Benefit-Risk Appraisal of Medicines

Benefit-Risk Appraisal of Medicines
A systematic approach to decision-making

Filip Mussen,
Johnson & Johnson Pharmaceutical Research and Development,
Beerse, Belgium

Sam Salek,
Cardiff University, Cardiff, UK

Stuart Walker,
CMR International Institute for Regulatory Science, London, UK

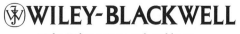
A John Wiley & Sons, Ltd., Publication

This edition first published 2009, © 2009 John Wiley & Sons, Ltd

Wiley-Blackwell is an imprint of John Wiley & Sons, formed by the merger of Wiley's global Scientific, Technical and Medical business with Blackwell Publishing.

Registered office: John Wiley & Sons Ltd, The Atrium, Southern Gate, Chichester, West Sussex, PO19 8SQ, UK

Other Editorial Offices:

9600 Garsington Road, Oxford, OX4 2DQ, UK

111 River Street, Hoboken, NJ 07030-5774, USA

For details of our global editorial offices, for customer services and for information about how to apply for permission to reuse the copyright material in this book please see our website at www.wiley.com/wiley-blackwell

Library of Congress Cataloging-in-Publication Data

Salek, Sam.
 Benefit-risk appraisal of medicines : a systematic approach to decision making /
Sam Salek, Stuart R. Walker, Filip Mussen.
  p. ; cm.
Includes bibliographical references and index.
ISBN 978-0-470-06085-8 (cloth)
1. Drugs—Testing. 2. Pharmaceutical policy—Decision making.
I. Walker, Stuart R., 1944– II. Mussen, Filip. III. Title.
[DNLM: 1. Drug Evaluation—standards. 2. Decision Support Techniques.
3. Models, Theoretical. 4. Risk Assessment. QV 771 S163b 2009]
RM301.27.S25 2009
615'.1901—dc22

                                                          2009019338

A catalogue record for this book is available from the British Library.

ISBN: 978-0-470-06085-8 (H/B)

Set in 10.5/13pt Times by Integra Software Services Pvt. Ltd, Pondicherry, India
Printed in Great Britain by CPI Antony Rowe, Chippenham, Wiltshire

First impression—2009

Contents

Foreword

Balancing benefits and risks forms an integral part of everyday life – personal, financial and professional; yet there is little agreement as to how this can be measured and expressed.

Take two clinical scenarios. First, a medicine has the potential to cure cancer or successfully treat a severe infection without causing major adverse effects; second a medicine is used for the treatment of transient muscle aches but causes frequent skin rashes. In each of these instances the benefit–risk balance is obvious. But most therapeutic options are not so easy and more often concern marginal benefits and risks which are difficult to assess. In addition, the same experimental information on risks and benefits of a new medicine may be interpreted differently by the drug developer, the regulator, the healthcare professional and the patient.

None of this is new. The lexicon of risk has been inconclusively debated for years and used differently by various stakeholders. What is lacking is a systematic approach to decision making and communication. In therapeutics the need for such an approach has never been greater. As powerful new medicines for hitherto untreatable diseases are produced, all concerned parties must decide whether their potential for benefit outweighs that for causing harm, and should be able to engage in a dialogue to express this.

Such an assessment is not only made at the time of application for marketing authorization of a new product. At each stage of the development process, both preclinical and clinical, risk and benefit are continually balanced. As more evidence accrues as on the effectiveness and safety of a medicine when it is in widespread clinical use, this balance may change markedly and require regulatory action, resulting in either allowing its more extensive use for new indications or in limiting its usage to specified groups of patients. The latter represents a special problem for the regulator. By restricting the use of a new medicine to a group of patients who, for example, may have already failed treatment with other therapeutic agents which may have resulted in impairment of an already compromised immune system, the regulator may cause the balance to swing against its further successful use. Formal assessment of the benefit risk balance and its clear communication by all parties involved in this situation would facilitate more informed debate.

But another party is assuming greater importance in the discussion surrounding benefit and risk. Approval by health technology assessors and reimbursers decides whether already financially pressed healthcare systems will allow a new drug to be widely used. Although such decisions are predominantly made on considerations of clinical and cost effectiveness, implicit in these is an appreciation of risk and benefit. The measurements used in health technology assessment differ from those of the developer and the regulator, but can be accommodated into various models, and these considerations are discussed in the text that follows.

This book provides a review of how present concepts of benefit and risk in the assessment of medicines have developed and how these are interpreted in various countries by various stakeholders. It describes a framework in which various models can be accommodated, illustrating these with important worked clinical examples. The authors have contributed to this field for many years and their ideas have been refined by workshops, discussions and debates reports of which are helpfully included as appendices to the book. This will not be the last word in a rapidly moving field but as an expression of the current state of the art, it has much to commend it.

Professor Sir Alasdair Breckenridge CBE
Chair of the Medicine Healthcare products
Regulatory Agency (MHRA)

Preface

This project began in the year 2000 as the result of increasing questions and challenges about the benefit-risk appraisal decisions by major regulatory agencies. This was originally intended for publication in the drug safety/pharmacoepidemiology literature. However, later it became evident that, given the continued debate and a greater need for a systematic, explicit and transparent approach to decision-making, to target the manuscript just at a limited audience would probably bypass the very groups who would benefit most from its message. Furthermore, the book is wider in its scope and includes the entire work of the project including its conceptualisation and rationale.

The book progressed in three phases: firstly an understanding of current practices of benefit-risk appraisal including the CIOMS recommendations and existing models; secondly, a review of benefit-risk appraisals in other industries and their approach to decision-making; and thirdly, the development of a new model for benefit-risk appraisal of medicines based on the multi-criteria decision analysis technique and the proposal of a future framework for benefit-risk appraisal of medicines.

In an attempt to openly debate these issues of concern to the pharmaceutical industry, regulatory authorities, practitioners and patients, the authors communicated their work and its practical application through a series of workshops and reports which are reflected as appendices in this book. The chapters are carefully selected to develop a systematic approach to the debate and at the same time to foster the way of thinking in order to make the book of interest to a wider audience. Moreover, the subject has a wide appeal and that coupled with the pioneering work presented by the authors should indisputably place this book next to an essential reading or reference list for the pharmaceutical industry and regulatory authorities worldwide as well as students pursuing postgraduate degrees in pharmacoepidemiology/pharmacovigilance, clinical research, pharmaceutical medicine, pharmacy and medicine.

We welcomed the opportunity of working together for the preparation of this book and thank the publishing team at John Wiley for their patience and understanding during the rather long preparation period for this book. Our thanks go to our families and friends for their support while this book was in preparation.

Filip Mussen
Sam Salek
Stuart Walker

CHAPTER 1

Concept and Scope of Benefit–Risk Evaluation of Medicines

1.1 HISTORICAL BACKGROUND

The regulation of modern medicines started after the thalidomide tragedy, which was undoubtedly the most significant adverse event in pharmaceutical history. It was a tragedy because the toxic effects of the medicine were expressed through the damage to the unborn foetus between the fortieth and fiftieth days of gestation after the mother had taken therapeutic doses of the medicine as a sedative or hypnotic during the pregnancy. The baby was born with characteristic reduction deformities of the limbs with shortening or complete absence of long bones, the hands and feet being attached as 'flippers' or absent altogether (Burley, 1988). The plight of these children, about 1000 who were born in the United Kingdom and several thousands in West Germany, caused widespread horror and emotional reactions and calls for all medicines to be the subject of governmental control and regulation in order to avoid a repetition of such an event.

A previous disaster in 1938, when 107 deaths were caused in the United States by the consumption of an 'elixir' of sulfanilamide containing a toxic solvent, had led to the setting up of new legislation in the United States whereby manufacturers of medicines had to be registered, had to carry out safety tests and were liable to receive factory inspections and seizure of products in violation (Burley, 1988). The thalidomide tragedy led to the strengthening of the regulatory process, particularly in respect of prescription medicines and the introduction of the requirement for pre-marketing submission to the regulatory authorities in the United States as well as in Europe.

Benefit-Risk Appraisal of Medicines   Filip Mussen, Sam Salek, Stuart Walker
© 2009 John Wiley & Sons, Ltd

Already in 1962, after the thalidomide tragedy had become known, MacGregor and Perry (1962) made the following very wise comments with regard to the impact of thalidomide on regulations worldwide:

> Such hazards can become apparent only on prolonged clinical use of drugs in human patients. Tragedies will no doubt continue to occur with new remedies, and this is part of the price to be paid for therapeutic progress, because we cannot, as a community, ask for new drugs without being prepared to accept such risks. We cannot legislate ourselves out of this dilemma . . .

Since 1962, a significant number of breakthrough medicines have been put on the market in a vast number of therapeutic areas such as hypertension, heart failure, hypercholesterolaemia, schizophrenia, cancer, human immunodeficiency virus (HIV), etc. The regulatory authorities have assessed all these products with regard to their quality, safety and efficacy, but the emphasis was usually put on the safety. Whenever Food and Drug Administration (FDA) Commissioners were called to testify before Congress, the charge was usually 'Why did you put this drug on the market which later turned out to be toxic?' It was not until the acquired immune deficiency syndrome (AIDS) epidemic surfaced that Congress began to ask the FDA why certain medicines were not on the market (Lasagna, 1998). The statement by the FDA (1999b) provides a very good and balanced perspective with regard to the benefits (efficacy) and risks (safety) of medicines: 'Although medical products are required to be safe, safety does not mean zero risk. A safe product is one that has reasonable risks, given the magnitude of the benefit expected and the alternatives available. All participants in the medical product development and delivery system have a role to play in maintaining this benefit–risk balance by making sure that products are developed, tested, manufactured, labelled, prescribed, dispensed, and used in a way that maximizes benefit and minimizes risk.'

The role of regulatory authorities is well defined in this respect, and regulatory authorities approve a new medicine or confirm approval of a marketed medicine when they judge that the benefits of using a medicine outweigh the risks for the intended population and use, and they ensure that the medicine is truthfully and adequately labelled for the population and use (Food and Drug Administration, 1999b). The key question is however *how* the regulatory authorities judge whether the benefits outweigh the risks, or in other words, how is the benefit–risk balance of a medicine established? This basic question triggered this book, also because it is recognized that balancing the benefits and risks is probably one of the most difficult tasks for anyone involved either in the development of new medicines or in the post-approval re-assessment of marketed medicines, and that basic research is still needed in this area (Edwards and Hugman, 1997). The next question is then whether methods, models or other tools have been developed or can be used to aid the regulatory authorities and others in determining the overall benefit–risk balance of medicines. Since the regulatory authorities are not the only stakeholder with regard to medicines, these questions should be considered in the context of how the other stakeholders (pharmaceutical companies, prescribers, and patients) judge whether the benefits of a medicine outweigh the risks.

An overview on benefit–risk assessment is provided in the next sections of this chapter. Following a review of the regulatory systems for assessing medicines, definitions, views and perceptions of benefits and risks will be outlined. Next, concepts as well as current practices in benefit–risk assessment will be discussed, and finally an overview on the use of methods and models for benefit–risk assessment will be provided.

1.2   THE REGULATORY SYSTEMS FOR ASSESSING MEDICINES

As outlined below, the concept of benefit versus risk is well captured in the EU and US legislation, which provide the legal framework for benefit–risk assessments by the regulatory authorities.

Europe

In the European Union, medicines must meet the three exclusive criteria laid down in the Community law which are quality, safety and efficacy, for a marketing authorization to be granted (Brunet, 1999). In Directive 2001/83/EC on the Community code relating to medicinal products for human use it is stipulated that a marketing authorization shall be refused if: (a) the risk–benefit balance is not considered to be favourable, or (b) its therapeutic efficacy is insufficiently substantiated by the applicant, or (c) its qualitative and quantitative composition is not as declared (Official Journal of the European Communities, 2004). Furthermore, in the preambles to this Directive, the following is stated:

> The concepts of harmfulness and therapeutic efficacy can only be examined in relation to each other and have only a relative significance depending on the progress of scientific knowledge and the use for which the medicinal product is intended. The particulars and documents which must accompany an application for marketing authorization for a medicinal product demonstrate that potential risks are outweighed by the therapeutic efficacy of the product.

As an example of the application of the EU regulations, in the United Kingdom the Committee on Safety of Medicines (CSM) looks for evidence of the medicine's safety, efficacy and quality when considering an application for a product licence. The CSM also uses benefit–risk analyses for medicines already licensed, and they have the right to change a license to minimize the risks from taking a medicine whilst allowing specific patients continuing benefit (Risk:benefit analysis of drugs in practice, 1995).

United States

The US drug law first embraced the idea of risk versus benefit in 1962. Providing evidence of safety before marketing was first required by the Federal Food, Drug and Cosmetic Act in 1938. However, it was not until the Kefauver–Harris Drug Amendments of 1962 that firms had to show a drug's effectiveness before marketing (FDA, 1999a). Today, the FDA decides before any medicine is marketed whether the studies submitted by the drug's sponsor show it to be safe and effective for its intended use. This decision comes down to two questions: (1) do the results of well-controlled studies provide substantial evidence of effectiveness? (2) do the results show that the product is safe under the condition of use in the proposed labelling (safe, in this context, means that the benefits of the drug appear to outweigh its risks) (FDA, 1999a)?

Japan

Similar to the EU and the United States, in Japan the quality, efficacy and safety of a medicine are assessed by the Ministry of Health and Welfare (Japan Pharmaceutical Manufacturers Association, 2003), and approval is an official confirmation that the medicine is both safe and effective (Danjoh, 1999).

The YUYOSEÏ instrument, which is required in Japanese clinical trials and which is a global assessment given by the physician to reflect an individual's overall response to a treatment, will be discussed later in this chapter.

1.3   BENEFIT–RISK ASSESSMENT: DEFINITIONS

Several authors have defined the words 'benefit' and 'risk', and some have proposed using other terms because in their view the term 'benefit–risk assessment' is incorrect.

According to Webster's Dictionary (1991), 'benefit' originates from the Latin words '*bene factum*' and means 'something that promotes well-being, advantage'. 'Risk' means 'possibility of loss or injury, peril' or 'a dangerous element or factor'. The FDA (2002) defined, in its information to consumers, benefits of medicines as 'helpful effects you get when you use medicines, such as lowering blood pressure, curing infection or relieving pain', and risks as 'the chances that something unwanted or unexpected could happen to you when you use medicines'. The WHO Collaborating Centre for International Drug Monitoring used similar definitions for benefit ('the proven therapeutic good of a product; should also include the patient's subjective assessment of its effects') and risk ('the probability of harm being caused; the probability (chance, odds) of an occurrence') (The Uppsala Monitoring Centre, 2002a).

An important difference between benefit and risk is that 'benefit' is a quantity (in preventive medicine, the magnitude of the loss or harm averted) whereas 'risk' is a probability (the likelihood of the occurrence of an unfavourable event) (Cheung and Kumana, 2001). In this respect, Cheung and Kumana argued that a minimal benefit can never be attractive, even if there is a 99% chance of gaining it. On the other hand, a tiny risk, say 1%, cannot always be ignored, especially if the penalty is something unpleasant. Similarly, Herxheimer (2001) stated that benefits and risks have completely different dimensions (a benefit is a material or experiential good thing, while a risk is a probability, the chance that something bad will happen), and that therefore 'benefit' should be weighed against 'harm', and the probability of benefit against the probability of harm. Veatch (1993) also mentioned that the proper contrasting terms are 'benefit' and 'harm', not benefit and risk. Edwards *et al.* (1996) went one step further and argued that the phrase 'benefit–risk' is clumsy and has been used in too many different contexts. The preferred term was therefore 'merit assessment' since it unambiguously indicates the determination of the worth of a medicine in a given context.

The term 'benefit–risk ratio' is used very often in the literature, but several authors have argued that this term is very often inaccurate. Herxheimer (2001) and Ernst and Resch (1996) stated that, because the benefit and the risk are not of the same nature, no one can really weigh them. Similarly, in the CIOMS IV report it was mentioned that for many benefit–risk assessments, neither the benefits nor the risks are easily or appropriately compared quantitatively (CIOMS Working Group IV, 1998). Hence, the word 'ratio', which is a mathematical term, is incorrectly used in this context (Edwards *et al.*, 1996). 'Benefit–risk balance' is a more general and therefore more appropriate term, which is used for example in the new EU pharmaceutical legislation and defined as 'an evaluation of the positive therapeutic effects of the medicinal product in relation to the risks', with risks being defined as 'any risk relating to the quality, safety and efficacy of the medicinal product as regards the health of patients' (Council of the European Union, 2003). The terms 'risk–benefit ratio' or 'risk–benefit assessment' are also sometimes used in the literature, although it can be argued that putting risks before benefits is inappropriate and that benefit–risk is a more logical order.

In this book, the terms 'benefit', 'risk' and 'benefit–risk balance' will be used preferentially because they are most frequently used in the literature and by regulatory authorities, despite the fact that it would be more accurate to use the term 'harm' instead of risk.

1.4   VIEWS AND PERCEPTIONS OF BENEFITS AND RISKS OF MEDICINES

Health care professionals' perspectives

In this section, the views and perceptions of the professionals involved in benefit–risk assessment, which are the pharmaceutical companies, the regulatory authorities, and prescribers will be described.

As a prerequisite, it is important to note that benefit and risk are fundamentally evaluative terms (Veatch, 1993). According to Veatch, they each contain in their very meaning value judgements that, in principle, cannot be made scientifically. Clinical studies, within the limits of their statistical power, can show that a medicine will have an effect. What studies cannot do is determine whether the effect is a benefit and, if so, how beneficial the effect is. Neither can they determine that the effect is a risk (harm) and, if so, how harmful. For example, the science can determine within certain limits what the change in 1-year survival probability is from the use of a medicine, but it cannot determine how valuable it is to survive. In this respect, it has been argued that providing information in terms of extension of lives instead of saving of lives would give a more realistic and balanced assessment of the efficacy of a medicine, and should moreover include an assessment of the quality and quantity of the life (Tan and Murphy, 1999). In general, the science can determine what the change in mortality rate is or what the cause of a rash is, but it cannot determine how bad it is for these events to occur (Veatch, 1993). In fact, it cannot even determine whether the effect is good or bad, that is, whether it is a benefit or a harm (risk). At the extreme, some people suffering from very serious conditions would count on a rapid painless drug-induced death a benefit rather than a harm. Still according to Veatch, benefit and risk (harm) are categories that necessarily involve subjective value judgements that ultimately only patients themselves can make, and this fact has radical implications for how information about benefit and risk judgements is processed by the regulatory authorities. Obviously judgements must be based on facts about what the effects of a medicine are likely to be. However, it requires superimposing evaluative judgements on these facts, and labelling the effects as good or bad, helpful or harmful. This requires drawing on religious, cultural, social and political judgements about how a medicine fits the basic values of society (Veatch, 1993). Veatch provides the example of two hypothetical medicines, one of which has a 50% success rate in curing its target disease but a 0.01% mortality rate. The other has a 60% success rate, but a 1% mortality rate. It is absolutely impossible to determine whether either of these medicines is safe or effective based on these data. If the medicines treat headaches, virtually everyone would make the value judgement that neither is safe enough nor, perhaps, effective enough neither. If the medicines are used to treat small cell lung carcinoma, perhaps both would be judged safe and effective enough to give patients the right to access, but what if these medicines treat a serious, occasionally fatal condition such as paranoid schizophrenia? This example shows clearly that weighing benefits and risks of a medicine is a value judgement. According to Rawlins (1987), comparing benefits and risks is the problem of comparing apples and pears, or of titrating for example one life saved versus 1000 patients with impotence. A complicating factor is often that long-term benefits have to be weighted against short term risks, or vice versa. For example, with the oral contraceptive pill a benefit of no fear of getting pregnant (tomorrow) must be compared with a risk of venous thrombosis or myocardial infarction (15 to 25 years in the future) (Herxheimer, 2001). However, most people are less concerned about an adverse event that might occur in the future compared with one that might occur in the present, a process known as 'discounting' (Naimark et al., 1997). In contrast, for a statin for the treatment of hypercholesterolaemia, the long-term benefit of a decreased risk of coronary heart disease must be weighted against the risk of adverse effects in the short-term such as myopathy. The time-dependence of benefit–risk has so far not been addressed appropriately (O'Neill, 2008).

Having established this fundamental concept of value judgement, the next question is how pharmaceutical companies, regulatory authorities and prescribers view benefits and risks of medicines. Pharmaceutical companies view benefits of medicines in terms of their ability to demonstrate sufficient efficacy so that: (1) regulatory authorities will approve their product, (2) third-party payers will reimburse for the medicine, (3) physicians will prescribe the medicine, and (4) people will purchase and use the medicine (Spilker, 1994). Risks are usually viewed as adverse experiences relative to existing treatment. Companies may accept increased risks until they reach the point where regulatory authorities will not approve, or physicians will not prescribe the medicine. Another driving force behind many risk assessments is legal liability (Bowen, 1993). Within a company some groups traditionally focus to a greater degree on potential risks (e.g. lawyers, research and development staff), while others tend to focus primarily on benefits (e.g. marketers, public relations, advertising staff).

Regulatory authorities tend to view benefits and risks for the nation as a whole rather than for individuals (Spilker, 1994; Cromie, 1987). Because of the cost of treatment to society and the required trade-offs that have to be made in this respect, this may lead to a conflict between the interests of individual patients and the population (Swales, 1997). Also, regulatory authorities evaluate the benefits and risks of a medicine against available alternatives (Bass, 1987; SCRIP, 2000), and they usually focus more on risks than benefits because of their mandate to protect society's health (Spilker, 1994). Just as the nature of the disease being treated is important for regulatory authorities in balancing benefits and risks of medicines, the purpose of the intervention will also impact the benefit–risk assessment (Arlett, 2001). Medicines may be used for prevention, treatment (symptomatic, curative, reduction of morbidity and/or mortality, stabilization, improvement of quality of life), or diagnosis. Regulatory authorities require a very well established and favourable safety profile for medicines used for the prevention of a disease, in particular if that disease is non-serious, and for medicines which treat symptoms (Miller, 1993). In general, regulators tend to view patients as incompetent to judge risks and benefits (Bowen, 1993). Finally, since benefit–risk assessment is essentially a value judgement, inevitably it will be prone to a number of biases. Some people who make individual decisions will be risk-prone while others will be risk-averse on a particular issue. Other people might well reach different decisions on another occasion, even when presented with the same data (Rawlins, 1987). According to Asscher (1986), a selection bias is inevitable because of the difficulty to digest all the evidence presented. For example, FDA Advisory Committee members review only a small fraction of documentation included in a New Drug Application, and most members are not provided with a formal training in the interpretation of toxicology data or other important aspects of a safety evaluation. Hence the mechanisms employed by Advisory Committee members to assess safety and efficacy are largely based on clinical judgement (Lewis, 1993).

Prescribers view the benefits of a medicine in relative terms. They assess or guess whether other doses, other medicines or a non-medicine treatment will enhance or reduce the degree or type of benefit obtained (Spilker, 1994). Risks may offset one another in that a medicine may increase risks of adverse experiences but lower risks attributable to the disease being treated (Spilker, 1994). However, sometimes the risks of a medicine are given greater emphasis by prescribers relative to the risks of the disease being treated because the prescriber feels causally responsible for the former (Edwards *et al.*, 1996). Overall, they discuss the benefits of treatment more than the risks, as shown in a study (Elwyn *et al.*, 2003). In this respect, it should also be noted that perceptions of benefits and risks by physicians are strongly influenced by the way the data are presented in scientific journals and advertisements (Skolbekken, 1998). Also, it is felt that whilst great progress has been made in obtaining reliable evidence on the beneficial effects of a treatment, reliable evidence on harms is often lacking (Cuervo and Clarke, 2003). Finally, several authors advocate that there should be more education of prescribers on the evaluation of benefits and risks of medicines (Edwards and Hugman, 1997; Risk:benefit analysis of drugs in practice, 1995). This need for more education can be illustrated by a statement with regard to the class of cyclo-oygenase-2 (COX-2) inhibitors, that it is still difficult to give patients an honest, accurate, and understandable account of the balance between their benefits (relief of pain and improved function) and risks (the likelihood of serious adverse effects) (Jones, 2002).

Patients' and the general public perspectives

In its guide to patients, the FDA advises patients that they must decide what risks they can and will accept to get the benefits of medicines they want. For example, in a life-threatening disease, they might choose to accept more risk in the hope of getting the benefits of a cure or living a longer live. On the other hand, if patients are facing a minor illness, they might decide that they want to take very little risk, although the FDA recognizes that the benefit–risk decision is sometimes difficult to make for patients (FDA, 2002). The FDA also advises on some specific ways for patients to lower the risks and obtain the full benefits of medicines: talk to the doctor and other health care professionals, know your medicines, read the label and follow directions, avoid inter-actions, and monitor the medicine's effect. Similarly, Lumpkin (2000) argues that the fundamental goal of risk education must be to help patients understand that it is not a question of risk alone, but of benefit–risk, and how health care professionals know about benefits and risks relates to the individual patient and the decisions he or she has to make regarding their personal health.

According to Spilker, patients view benefits in terms of whether their symptoms improve, by how much and for how long. For medicines that prevent or suppress a disease or problem, benefits are viewed as how well they accomplish those goals. Risks are viewed as the likelihood of having adverse reactions, exacerbations or new episodes of the underlying disease, or other medicine-related problems. Risks that a patient voluntarily accepts (e.g. smoking cigarettes, using oral contraceptives) are often differentiated from those where little or no choice is possible (e.g. cosmic radiation) (Spilker, 1994). In addition, patients often have the misconception that medicines should be completely safe, which may lead them to focus excessively on any risks to which their attention is drawn. Perception of risk may therefore be different from actual risk (Edwards et al., 1996). Most people knowingly accept risk if (1) the probability of something harmful happening is small or distant in time, or (2) the possible harmful event is not serious, or (3) the possible benefits are sufficiently strong. For each person this kind of risk assessment is different and each person applies different criteria to different kinds of risks. AIDS patients have different views on what they perceive to be an acceptable risk compared to what regulatory authorities and industry perceive to be acceptable (Bowen, 1993). Perception of risk is affected by many variables from the tiny workings of individual psychology through the sweeping influences of language and culture (The Uppsala Monitoring Centre, 2002b). Overall, patients' perspectives on assessing benefits and risks are not by any means uniform. They often realize that benefits and harms necessarily require very personal, subjective value judgements that can only be based on religious, philosophical, and social values (Veatch, 1993). In a study by Johnson et al. (1994), women's views on the benefits and risks of hormone replace-ment therapy were measured using utility analysis. Results showed that women are reluctant to accept any increase in a risk factor such as a small increase in the risk of breast cancer, even if it reduces their total risk (which includes cardiovascular disease, osteoporosis, uterine cancer, ovarian cancer, breast cancer). A social climate, which is increasingly intolerant of risk, has created a tendency to seek absolute safety and security. This has led to a trend of blaming and punishing those who are seen to be the cause of accident or misadventure. Part of this results from an unwillingness to accept that it is natural for accidents to happen, and that there is always some uncertainty in all human activities, in spite of legislation or good intentions. Part of it results from the pressure on politicians and public servants to show that they are in control of the variables of existence (The Uppsala Monitoring Centre, 2002b).

Many factors influence patients' choices about treatment and its benefits and risks. These include their own attitudes and beliefs, as discussed above, and those expressed in the media, by other health professionals and by family and friends. Previous experience, trust in their physician and the chances of success also affect their decisions (Risk:benefit analysis of drugs in practice, 1995). Finally, perceptions of benefits and risks by patients are strongly influenced by the way the data are presented, which is also the case for physicians (Skolbekken, 1998). However, research has demonstrated that, despite the fact that lay people sometimes lack certain information about hazards, their basic conceptualization of risk is much 'richer' than that of the experts and reflects legitimate concerns that are typically omitted from expert risk assessments (Slovic, 1987).

A survey, whose purpose it was to establish whether patient groups across the EU considered that pharmaceutical companies should provide the public with more information on prescription medicines, revealed that the majority of patients are no longer willing to rely on doctors as the most important source of information about their prescription medicines (PatientView, 2002). Patients prefer a range of information sources about medicines, and the ideal source of information would be, amongst many other features, striking a balance between a treatment's beneficial and adverse effects (Dickinson and Raynor, 2003). Patients often desire more information than is currently provided, and professionals need to support patients in making choices by turning raw data into information that is more helpful to the discussions than the data (Edwards et al., 2002). Patients do not want to know all undesirable effects of a medicine, but only those which are relevant to them (Meiners, 2002). Overall, given the difficulties and ramifications of benefit–risk assessment, the challenge of presenting understandable, coherent information to patients is considerable (Edwards and Hugman, 1997). Similarly, regulatory authorities have difficulties in communicating information on benefit–risk assessments to patients because of a lack of information (Beermann, 2002). In this respect, Edwards made a number of recommendations with regard to communication of benefit–risk assessments to patients, and called for increased attention to more transparent, accurate and helpful benefit–risk assessments and expressions.

All of this is, however, to a certain extent in contrast with how the media cover the benefits and risks of medicines. In a study, coverage by US news media of the benefits and risks of three medicines that are used to prevent major diseases was analysed. The medicines were pravastatin (a cholesterol-lowering medicine for the prevention of cardiovascular disease), alendronate (a bisphosphonate for the treatment and prevention of osteoporosis) and aspirin (which is used for the prevention of cardiovascular disease). A systematic probability sample of 180 newspaper articles (60 for each medicine) and 27 television reports that appeared between 1994 and 1998 were analysed. Of the 207 stories, 83 (40%) did not report benefits quantitatively. Of the 124 that did, 103 (83%) reported relative benefits only, 3 (2%) absolute benefits only, and 18 (15%) both absolute and relative benefits. Of the 207 stories, 98 (47%) mentioned potential harm to patients. It was concluded that news-media stories about medications may include inadequate or incomplete information about the benefits and risks about the medicines (Moynihan *et al.*, 2000). Moreover, it can be assumed that the vast majority of the intended audience will not take the time to read a full article as would be required to accurately understand the complex balance of benefit and risk (Califf, 2004). Other studies had identified an overstatement of adverse effects and risks, with negative clinical trials being highlighted and positive trials being ignored (Lebow, 1999), and that media coverage was driven by moral outrage instead of scientific notions of calculable risk (Brown *et al.*, 1996). Yet another study came to a somewhat different conclusion that in the Netherlands a discrepancy exists between the medical literature and the newspapers, in that the negative consequences of the use of medicines receive proportionally more attention in the professional literature than in the newspapers, whilst this difference does not exist for 'good news' (van Trigt *et al.*, 1995).

1.5 STAGES AND CONCEPTS IN BENEFIT–RISK ASSESSMENT

When is benefit–risk assessment used?

Benefit–risk assessment is used during the various stages of the life cycle of a medicine: during the development of a new medicine, during the approval phase of a new medicine, and for the post-approval re-assessment of marketed medicines. A short description of how benefit–risk assessment is used during these three stages is provided below.

Benefit–risk assessment during the development of a new medicine

The safety and efficacy profile of a new medicine gradually takes shape over the course of the development of a new medicine, but will not even be fully elucidated by the time that the medicine finishes its development. Also, whilst during the early stages of development more weight is placed on the animal data because these are essentially the only data available, human experience becomes more important as development progresses (Brimblecombe, 1987). The major technique for incorporating benefit–risk considerations during the development stage is through the use of minimally acceptable hurdles (Spilker, 1994). These standards specifically identify the types and magnitudes of activities the compound must have (or must not have) at each stage of the development to further progress. The rationale for the creation of these hurdles, which are essentially benefit and risk hurdles, is that unless a compound meets the minimum standards, there is little or no reason to continue its development. An important factor in this respect is that a company that is developing a new medicine may be unaware of a competitor who has a safer or more effective medicine under development. Introduction of a major competitive product can instantly turn what might have been an important advance in therapy into a product that will not be approved by a regulatory authority or will not be widely prescribed.

Specifically, benefit–risk assessment is initially considered of importance during the phase II dose-ranging studies in selecting the dose or doses for the phase III trials, based on a trade-off of the efficacy and safety observed with each dose. As will be discussed in the next section, some models exist for this purpose. Obviously the phase III data offer the best chance to conduct a meaningful benefit–risk assessment prior to the market entry of the medicine, and they are the basis for the benefit–risk assessment by the regulatory authorities as discussed below. Nevertheless, at least one author suggests that benefit–risk assessment in the development of a new medicine is often done on an *ad hoc* basis, and there are few cases where the user of the phrase was specific about how this assessment should be conducted (Chuang-Stein, 1999).

Benefit–risk assessment during the approval process of a new medicine

Decisions on the benefit–risk balance of a new medicine by regulatory authorities are generally speaking based on the legislation in place, which is comparable throughout the Western world (Bass, 1987). Nevertheless, different regulatory authorities can come to different decisions based on the same data, and this is because of differences in administrative and scientific views and interpretations. In addition, regulatory authorities have to make decisions based on incomplete data, with more safety and efficacy data becoming available during the commercialiation of the medicine. Also, they compare a new medicine with the available alternatives (Bass, 1987), and although not published, the EU Committee for Human Medicinal Products (CHMP) has made it clear that they would not approve a medicine which has a benefit–risk profile which is inferior to existing therapy.

According to Chuang-Stein (1999), benefit–risk assessment remains largely a concept rather than a routine practice in the current regulatory environment. Even though everyone agrees on the need to conduct such an assessment, few can come up with the specifics to actually carry it out. Miller (1992) cited the lack of attention paid to the benefit–risk issues as one pitfall that frequently delays the review and approval process. Nevertheless, pharmaceutical companies rarely receive any guidance from the regulatory authorities regarding the basics and contents of a pertinent benefit–risk assessment package (Miller, 1992; Chuang-Stein, 1999). Walker stated in the mid-1980s that as a result of a more accurate assessment of benefits and risks in the next 10 or 20 years, it may be possible to plot on a matrix system (Figure 1.1) any new chemical entity at the approval stage, or at the post-approval stage (Walker, 1987). Whilst there is no hard evidence that the benefit–risk assessments of new medicines conducted today are superior to the assessments made in the eighties, the basic matrix proposed by Walker is still valid. More recently, it was suggested that the emerging risk management strategies including extensive and earlier epidemiological assessments of benefits and risks of new medicines will eventually create a new standard of evidence for industry and regulators (Andrews and Dombeck, 2004).

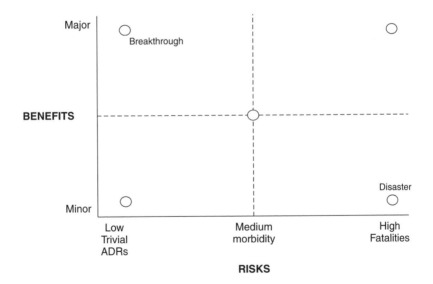

Figure 1.1   Matrix system for plotting the benefit–risk ratio of medicines

Finally, it should be noted that cost-benefit assessment is not part of the approval process of new medicines either in Europe or in the United States. Costs and health economics in a broader sense are not considered during the approval process of new medicines.

Benefit–risk assessment during the post-approval re-assessment of marketed medicines

At the time medicines are initially approved by the regulatory authorities, evidence for the efficacy and safety will have been more or less secured. However, at that stage, efficacy has often only been established in a limited number of patients under a narrow range of conditions, and safety in relatively small number of patients. During the post-marketing period, evidence may accumulate to suggest that the efficacy is considerable in a wider group of patients than was originally indicated or that the medicine has a true impact on clinical outcomes as opposed to surrogate outcomes, and that safety during long-term use in a more heterogeneous population is acceptable. Alternatively, efficacy may appear to be less satisfactory than originally believed and safety becomes pre-judiced (Rawlins, 1987). The UK Committee on Safety of Medicines considered that the following issues might lead to changes in the benefit–risk profile of a marketed medicine (Rawlins, 1987):

1. quality (very unusual)

2. efficacy

    (a) new evidence for lack of efficacy

    (b) uniqueness of therapeutic properties

    (c) uniqueness of efficacy in small patient subgroups

3. safety

    (a) spontaneous reports

        literature

        yellow cards

        other agencies

    (b) cohort studies

    (c) case–control studies

    (d) animal carcinogenicity.

Apart from the new information about the medicine itself, external factors not involving the medicine may change the benefit–risk balance (Spilker, 1994). These include the introduction of new medicines, combination therapy or other modalities that compete with the original medicine.

Following the benefit–risk assessment of a marketed medicine based on new information, it will sometimes be necessary to take action either to increase the benefit of the medicine by improving its rational use, or reducing the risk usually by restricting its use (Arlett, 2001). With regard to the latter, formal risk management plans are now being established for new medicines, which aim at minimizing the risks while maximizing the beneficial effects of a medicine by ensuring its proper use by the right patients for the right disease conditions (Marwick, 1999; Perfetto *et al.*, 2003). If the overall balance of benefits and risks is judged to be negative, then the medicine may be withdrawn unless risk reduction strategies can be identified which would swing the balance away from risk. In this respect, the following actions may be taken (Arlett, 2001):

- continue to passively monitor the issue: may be appropriate for non-serious adverse events where causality is not established

- actively collect further data: if causality is not established, mechanism unclear, risk factors not identified

- add warnings to the product label: for less serious adverse effects, particularly those that are unavoidable, warning health care professionals and patients may be the only action necessary

- changes to the product label to reduce risk: restrict the indication, contraindicate those at greatest risk, advice monitoring

- monitor effects of action taken: ensure that the action effectively protects public health.

Concepts in benefit–risk assessment

Based on the above, a number of concepts and rules with regard to benefit–risk assessment and benefit–risk balance can be identified, all of which are also discussed in the literature, and some of which (concepts 3 and 4) are related to the fundamental paradigm that benefit–risk assessment and balance are value judgements, as discussed above.

Concept 1: a separate benefit–risk balance for each indication

It is generally recognized that a separate benefit–risk assessment should be conducted for each indication, because medicines are clinically tested for each indication separately (Spilker, 1994; Beckmann, 1999). The efficacy and thus the benefits of a medicine in one indication are not the same as in another indication, and, similarly, the safety is not necessarily comparable, one of the reasons being that the dosage might be different in different indications.

Concept 2: all available data should be considered in benefit–risk assessment

Several authors emphasize the need that all available and relevant data should be considered in benefit–risk assessment (Bass, 1987; Arlett, 2001). For example, an application to the regulatory authorities for a new medicine must include very comprehensive data and information with regard to the quality of the active and inactive substances and the finished product, the non-clinical studies (animal pharmacology and pharmacokinetics, animal toxicology including single and repeat-dose toxicity, genotoxicity, carcinogenicity, reproductive and developmental toxicity), and the clinical studies (human pharmacokinetic and pharmacodynamic studies, clinical efficacy and safety studies, and post-marketing experience if applicable) (International Conference on Harmonization, 2000). Thus, benefit–risk assessment involves the review and interpretation of a wealth of safety and efficacy information, which must eventually be captured in the benefit–risk balance.

Concept 3: the nature of the disease should be taken into account for benefit–risk balance

The seriousness and prognosis of the disease being treated by the medicine under investigation will have a major impact on the benefit–risk balance (Meyboom and Egberts, 1999; Schiller and Johnson, 2008). For example, if the disease is self-limiting such as influenza in an otherwise healthy young adult, serious adverse effects would be likely to result in a negative balance of benefits and risks. In contrast, with a disease with a high mortality, serious adverse effects may still be outweighed by the benefits afforded by the medicine (Arlett, 2001). In general, the more severe the disease, the more tolerable are the potential therapy risks (Miller, 1993). From a conceptual perspective, the seriousness of the disease can be compensated for in the evaluation of the benefits and/or risks, as suggested above, or alternatively the seriousness of the disease can be taken into account using the paradigm that the less severe the disease, the more the benefits of a medicine should outweigh its risks.

Concept 4: absolute versus relative benefit–risk balance

There seems to be a consensus in the literature that the availability of alternative therapies should be considered in benefit–risk assessment, and that the interpretation of the benefits and risks always involves a comparison (Bass, 1987; Miller, 1993; Spilker, 1994; Arlett, 2001). For example, the German Drug Law requires consideration of alternative sources of risk, namely: (1) the risk associated with no treatment, and (2) the benefit–risk balance of therapeutic alternatives, if available (Schosser, 2002). The US Federal Regulations do not require that new therapies be superior to or safer than existing therapies (nor do the EU regulations). The experience to date shows, however, that the best case for approval of a new medicine is where the disease is severe and/or life-threatening and for which there are few or no available treatments. This contrasts with the case for a medicine for which alternative therapies exist and for which lingering questions surrounding the safety of medicines in the therapeutic class remain unresolved (Miller, 1993). For example, according to the FDA the benefits of the diabetes compound Rezulin (troglitazone) outweighed its risks at the time of initial approval, but the launch of newer products with better safety profiles had made Rezulin 'outmoded' (SCRIP, 2000). In most cases benefit–benefit and risk–risk comparisons are made between the medicine in question and: (1) a higher or lower dose of the same medicine; (2) another medicine of the same type; (3) a medicine of a different type; (4) a combination of two or more medicines; (5) another treatment modality; or (6) a combination of a medicine plus another treatment modality (Spilker, 1994). As will be discussed in Chapter 2, pivotal clinical trials which aim at establishing the efficacy and safety profile of a new medicine include quite often an active comparator, and hence the comparison of the benefits and risks versus the alternative treatment is inherently part of the evaluation of the results of such trials. Thus, from the above it can be concluded that the benefit–risk balance is a relative and not an absolute concept.

Concept 5: the benefit–risk balance is dynamic and evolves over time

An important concept which is mentioned by many authors in the literature is that the benefit–risk balance is dynamic and changes over time (Rawlins, 1987; Spilker, 1994; Schosser, 2002; Konstam, 2003). The benefit–risk balance evolves as new information becomes available during the development of a new medicine, and the conclusions on the benefit–risk profile by the regulatory authorities at the time of market introduction of a new medicine may change after the medicine is marketed. With regard to the latter situation, the benefit–risk balance may change for two major categories of reasons. Those categories are: (1) new information about the medicine itself, and (2) external factors not involving the medicine (Spilker, 1994). Factors external to a medicine that affect its benefit–risk balance, as explained above in concept 4, include the introduction of new medicines, combination therapy or other modalities that compete with the medicine in question. In addition, the discovery of new problems with existing therapy may improve the benefit–risk balance of a new medicine.

The other reason for changes in the benefit–risk balance of a marketed medicine is new information about the medicine itself, which may lead to either increased or decreased benefits and/or risks. Increased risks occur regularly and are, for example, due to the appearance of new, rare side effects, or to a deterioration of the safety profile in populations with co-morbidities and/or concomitant medications which were not studied in the clinical development programme. An amelioration of the risk profile of a marketed medicine can also occur, an example being the demonstration in the Vioxx Gastrointestinal Outcomes Research (VIGOR) trial of significantly fewer clinically important upper gastrointestinal events with the COX-2 inhibitor rofecoxib than with naproxen (Bombardier *et al.*, 2000), although later the increased risk for cardiovascular effects became apparent. Similarly, the benefit of a marketed medicine may be reduced based on the results of new studies. For example, the angiotensin II antagonist losartan was originally approved in a number of countries for the treatment of heart failure based on the results of the Evaluation of Losartan in the Elderly (ELITE) trial, but the subsequent ELITE II trial showed that all-cause mortality (which was the primary endpoint of the trial) was numerically higher in patients treated with losartan than in patients treated with the angiotensin-converting enzyme (ACE) inhibitor captopril, which is standard treatment (Pitt *et al.*, 2000). There is also an inverse example in the field of congestive heart failure. Enalapril, an ACE inhibitor, which was originally approved for the treatment of heart failure based on exercise-tolerance studies only, was shown in the Studies of Left Ventricular Dysfunction (SOLVD) trial to reduce mortality and hospitalizations for heart failure (The SOLVD Investigators, 1991).

Schosser (2002) developed a decision matrix (Table 1.1) to determine the need for taking regulatory action in response to a change in the benefit–risk balance of a medicine. Classifying the change of either the risk or the benefit into one of the three categories 'increased', 'unchanged', or 'decreased' resulted in a 3×3 decision matrix. According to Schosser, action has to be taken whenever the benefit–risk balance falls below 'the bounds considered justifiable in the light of the knowledge of medical science', such as in the scenarios of increased risk with reduced or unchanged benefit, and reduced benefit with unchanged risk.

Table 1.1 Decision matrix to determine the need for taking regulatory action in response to a change of the benefit–risk balance of a medicine

Benefit	Risk		
	Reduced	Unchanged	Increased
Reduced	Conditional	Yes	Yes
Unchanged	No	No	Yes
Increased	No	No	Conditional

1.6   BENEFIT–RISK ASSESSMENT: THE CURRENT REGULATORY ENVIRONMENT

The withdrawal of the lipid-lowering medicine Baycol (cerivastatin) in 2001 and the withdrawal of the COX-2 inhibitor Vioxx (rofecoxib) in 2004 have drawn the increased attention of the stakeholders such as patients and physicians and the media to the regulatory processes for approving new medicines and for re-assessing marketed medicines. These two withdrawals raised major questions about the assessment of the safety of medicines and thus about their benefit–risk profile. Whilst the withdrawal of cerivastatin because of a non-acceptable risk for rhabdomyolysis was in many aspects different from the voluntary withdrawal of rofecoxib because of an increased risk of myocardial infarction after long-term use, both triggered the regulatory authorities to take a more cautious and conservative approach with regard to the safety and risk of medicines.

1.7   BENEFIT–RISK ASSESSMENT IN OTHER DISCIPLINES

Apart from the specific benefit–risk evaluations, benefits and risks of medicines are also considered, in addition to costs, in cost–benefit analysis and cost-effectiveness analysis. Cost–benefit analysis is considered the pre-eminent method of economic evaluation of medicines because it allows for the direct comparison of different types of outcomes resulting from a variety of actions (Messonnier and Meltzer, 2003). It provides the most comprehensive monetary measures of the positive (beneficial) and negative (costly) consequences of a possible course of action, such as recommending the routine vaccination of restaurant employees against hepatitis A. Because the results of cost–benefit analysis are expressed in monetary terms, both health and non-health programmes can be directly compared. Cost–benefit analysis has a long history in the study of environmental effects and natural resource use in the United States. Cost-effectiveness analysis has become the predominant method for evaluating the costs and effects of alternative health-care strategies (Gift *et al.*, 2003). It is a method used to evaluate the relationship between net investment and health improvement in health-care strategies competing for similar resources. Because cost-effectiveness analysis is limited to the comparison of strategies designed to improve health, no attempt is made to assign a monetary value to disease averted beyond the cost of care for persons with these conditions and costs of lost productivity from morbidity and mortality. Rather, results are presented in the form of the net cost per health outcome, such as 'cost per case prevented' or 'cost per life saved'. The decision-maker is left to make value judgements about the intrinsic value of the health outcomes. Cost-effectiveness analyses are designed to produce a cost-effectiveness ratio, the most commonly used summary measure for comparing health interventions (Gift *et al.*, 2003). The numerator of the cost-effectiveness ratio is the cost of the health intervention (including costs of adverse effects of the intervention and other costs induced by the intervention) minus the costs of the health conditions that are prevented as a result of the intervention. The denominator is the improvement in health produced by the intervention. This improvement in health may be measured in natural units, for example cases of measles prevented, or in terms of the impact on health-related quality of life, for example quality-adjusted life years. Cost-effectiveness analysis is becoming very important as new medicines must increasingly show evidence of cost-effectiveness before obtaining reimbursement. Faced with increasing health-care costs, the reimbursement authorities in many countries are now requiring proof of cost-effectiveness, the so-called fourth hurdle (Taylor *et al.*, 2004). It seems that these fourth hurdle policies are contributing to more cost-effective use of medicines.

In the health care sector, benefit–risk assessment is also applied to medical devices. Securing FDA approval of a new device before marketing requires that the manufacturer provides reasonable assurance that the device is safe and effective when used for the purpose for which the approval is sought (Kessler *et al.*, 1987). Safety and effectiveness are assessed with specific reference to the uses for which the device is intended, as detailed in the labelling on the device. Safety is evaluated by weighing the probable benefits to health against the probable risks of injury. The benefit–risk ratio must be acceptable, but proof that the product will never cause injury or will always be effective is not required. Similar regulations exist in Europe.

Benefit–risk assessments are also made in a vast number of fields outside the health care sector, although they are usually called risk assessments. They are rather widely applied with regard to energy (nuclear power, non-nuclear electric power), transport (motor vehicles, motorcycles, railways and aviation), food (e.g. the use of preservatives and colouring agents), sport activities (e.g. skiing, mountain climbing), and the environment (e.g. the use of pesticides) (Lee, 1987). In a number of these assessments, risks to human health are predominant. The problems and issues in such risk assessments are quite similar to the issues identified in this chapter for the benefit–risk assessment of medicines, the most important being that it is necessary to consider all benefits and all risks, and not only one aspect of the safety data in isolation (Alexander, 2002; CropLife International, 1997). Other issues that were for example identified for pesticides were that benefit–risk assessments are complex, and that it is inappropriate to undertake a comparative benefit–risk evaluation between two products when both products meet the acceptable standards for approval. Decision analysis techniques such as decision trees, Bayesian statistics, Monte Carlo simulations and sensitivity analyses are frequently used to make risk assessments (Clemen, 1996).

1.8 SPECIFIC METHODS AND MODELS FOR BENEFIT–RISK ASSESSMENT

Having described in the previous sections of this chapter the issues and difficulties with regard to benefit–risk assessment as well as the lack of guidance and standardization in this field, the purpose of this section is to provide a general overview of the possible methods and models for benefit–risk assessment that have been described and/or are being used by one or more stakeholders.

Definition of models and their potential value

Patten and Lee (2002) describe a model as 'something that mimics relevant features of a system being studied'. Models can assist with decision-making in a descriptive, heuristic or prescriptive (i.e. identifying optimal choices) sense. A model need not involve mathematical calculations. For example, a roadmap or a geological map can be regarded, by this definition, as a model. In fact, such non-mathematical models are often useful in decision making to clarify issues. However, explicit and analytic representation of a system usually requires a mathematical model. According to Patten and Lee a mathematical model can be defined as 'an abstract, simplified, mathematical construct related to a part of reality and created for a particular purpose'. Models can be used to simulate outcomes under a specified set of assumptions, and to help identify those factors, out of many possible factors, that may have the biggest impact on the outcome. Another advantage of a model is that it can be used to identify the degree to which changes in one or more variables impact the predicted output, which is called sensitivity analysis.

Back in 1985, Walker (1987) stated that the methodology for determining benefit–risk ratios was yet to be fully defined. He added that in the next 10 or 20 years, a stage may be reached when benefits could be accurately assessed, and that better ways and means of determining risks had to be found. More recently, it is still recognized that clinicians, members of formulary and guideline committees, and regulators must try to be much more specific when considering the benefits of treatments and the kinds of harm they may do (Herxheimer, 2001). If health care professionals can explain to each other how they weigh up the pluses and minuses for a particular intervention, then they will also be able to explain and discuss them more clearly and easily with patients. Medical judgement and consensus would have to be built into a methodology for benefit–risk assessment (Schosser, 2002). Since actual decisions concerning the balance between benefits and risks are heavily influenced by the values of the decision makers and difficult to quantify, better methods are needed for quantifying the benefit–risk profile and expressing the values involved in decision making (Hyslop *et al.*, 2002). Asscher (1986) mentioned four reasons why benefit–risk analysis assumes greater importance than in the past and why further improvement in the decision-making process is required:

1. Modern treatment more often concerns marginal benefits. The more marginal the gain, the more important to undertake benefit–risk analysis.

2. The modern therapeutic armamentarium contains many bolder forms of intervention, both medical and surgical. Partly as the result of the wise use of these, the population, now exposed to these more dangerous treatments, is older than it used to be. As also mentioned by Hyslop *et al.*, in the last 50 years medical science and especially pharmaceutical science has made tremendous progress, dramatically expanding the physician's therapeutic armamentarium. These advances bring the need to be more adept at assessing the benefit–risk balance, from the perspective of both society (the ill population) and the individual patient (Hyslop *et al.*, 2002).

3. Medical litigation is growing, and every decision in medicine involves a benefit–risk analysis which may have to stand up to critical examination by peers, patients, relatives, media and the courts.

4. Objective analysis of benefits and risks plays a pivotal role in regulatory decisions about medicines.

The use of decision analysis techniques has been advocated in the literature for medical decision-making in general, including benefit–risk assessments. Such decision-analytic models should be simple, because the insights derived from a simple model are similar to those derived from a complex formulation (Detsky *et al.*, 1997). To determine the appropriate level of complexity, it must be considered whether the model captures the key issues necessary to fully describe the benefit–risk trade-off. If a key element of the benefit–risk trade-off is missing, the model will not achieve its goal of helping to understand the trade-off. The potential advantages of a formal model based on decision-analysis techniques are as follows (Waller and Evans, 2003):

- increased transparency
- making reasoning explicit, reflecting complexity
- clearly identifying limitations of the evidence and uncertainty
- the impact of all assumptions can be assessed
- better justified decisions.

In the next sections, not only models for benefit–risk assessment will be reviewed, but also any other specific methods for benefit–risk assessment, the term 'method' being somewhat broader than the term 'model'.

Use of models in the literature

The question addressed in this section is whether in articles in scientific journals that review a specific medicine or a specific clinical trial, methods or models are used to describe the benefit–risk profile of the medicine in question. Whilst it would be outside the scope of this book to provide a complete overview of how benefit–risk assessments are described in the scientific literature, the focus of this review will be on scientific journals which specialize in benefit–risk assessment.

The journal *Drug Safety* is the premier international review journal covering the disciplines of pharmacovigilance, pharmacoepidemiology and benefit–risk assessment, and has a Scientific Citation Index Factor of 3.536 (Adis International, 2009). Since, according to the publisher, this journal includes benefit–risk assessments which provide an in-depth review of adverse effects and efficacy data for a medicine in a specific disease to place the benefit–risk relationship in clear perspective, it is of value to review how such benefit–risk assessments are made. For this purpose, all articles published between 1998 and 2002 and which included the terms 'benefit' and 'risk' in the title were reviewed with regard to the presence of a specific method to conduct the benefit–risk assessment. A search revealed that there were 48 articles that fitted these criteria, and that these articles pertained to benefit–risk assessments of specific medicines (24), specific classes of medicines (9), and medicines for specific diseases (15). The title of most of these articles was called 'A benefit–risk assessment of . . .' or 'A risk–benefit assessment of . . .'. From a review of these articles the following was concluded:

- whilst the efficacy and safety data were extensively reviewed in all articles, this review was not systematically extended and extrapolated into a discussion of the benefits and risks

- no systematic trade-off of the benefits and risks was performed

- overall, no systematic method for benefit–risk assessment was used in these articles, and the content and format of the specific sections of these articles which focused on the benefit–risk profile was not harmonized.

A recent review confirmed the previous findings.

In contrast to the above, Bjornson (2004) conducted a systematic review of the literature and came to the conclusion that the measurement of benefits and risks is consistently reported with similar terminology. However, he also concluded that the interpretation and subsequent balancing of benefits and risks was more problematic.

Use of models by pharmaceutical industry in drug development

Pharmaceutical companies use benefit–risk weighting in the drug development process. During earlier phases of drug development, research concentrates not only on dose-response modelling and identification of the maximally tolerated dose, but also on risk estimation for dose-dependent toxicity (Troche *et al.*, 2000). The goal is to find a dose that satisfies both safety and efficacy requirements. A simple method to obtain trade-off information is to specify, a priori, the maximum toxicity rate that would be acceptable if the new treatment were to produce 100% response, and similarly to specify a minimum response rate that would be acceptable if the treatment produced no toxicities (Conaway and Petroni, 1996). This method, in which the efficacy–toxicity requirements are specified, against which the medicines are then compared, can be applied to dose-finding studies and for other phase I and phase II trials.

There is a lack of available techniques during the drug development process to conduct relevant benefit–risk assessments to determine the acceptability of a new medicine across the dose range used in the therapeutic setting (Miller, 1992). Chuang-Stein (1994) developed a risk-adjusted benefit measure in which the intensity of side effects is quantified through a set of scores that are summarized into the risk component experienced by the individual. This approach of subtracting a multiple constant of the weighted risk component from the expected crude benefit is further described in Chapter 3.

Measurement of patient well-being and preference has become a focus of research in the area of clinical decision making (Troche *et al.*, 2000). Much of this work is motivated by the observation that increased attention to patients' quality of life results in greater levels of adherence to medication, satisfaction, and conformance to the principle of informed consent. The Committee for Medicinal Products for Human Use (CHMP) issued a reflection paper on the use of health-related quality-of-life (HRQL) measures in the evaluation of new medicines, which hinted at the increasing importance of such HRQL measures in randomized clinical trials and in the approval of new medicines (Committee for Medicinal Products for Human Use, 2004). One approach, q-TWiST (Quality-adjusted Time Without Symptoms of disease and Toxicity of treatment), is a method that compares therapies in terms of achieved survival and quality-of-life outcomes (Gelber *et al.*, 1996). Q-TWiST assesses both the likelihood of a given health state and the quality weighting to be assigned to that state. The result is a preference measure that captures both quality of life and time-linked data along a single index (Martin *et al.*, 1996).

Another approach is based on the multi-attribute utility theory (MAUT), a method that is founded on the theory of choice under uncertainty (Clemen, 1996). MAUT provides a quantifiable summary score and uses all available information on every defined, attainable health state (Troche *et al.*, 2000). MAUT permits direct comparisons across health interventions and even across therapeutic classes. For example, Eriksen and Keller (1993) developed a MAUT function to combine preferences for efficacy and toxicity of a medicine, and applied it to the evaluation of anti-glaucoma treatment. Their model is further mentioned in Chapter 3.

Another method, the probability trade-off technique (PTT), also emerges from the theory of choice. PTT involves a search for thresholds of indifference (Llewellyn-Thomas *et al.*, 1996). Descriptive and probabilistic information about potential benefits and side effects of two therapeutic alternatives are presented to patients and a point is located where the patient is indifferent between the two options. The method can determine how much benefit patients would require to accept a new therapy, which carries a particular risk of toxicity over an existing therapeutic intervention (Troche *et al.*, 2000). The resultant scale provides a relative measure of respondents' strength of preference for one option over another (Naylor and Llewellyn-Thomas, 1994). Troche *et al.* developed such a patient-specific drug safety-efficacy index to choose a specific therapeutic intervention and dosage, when known risks and benefits are reconciled against patient-specific preferences among an array of therapeutic alternatives. Their method is briefly discussed in Chapter 3.

All the above models measure the benefit and risk components using individual patient data, making benefit–risk trade-offs for individual patients. A few other models have been developed as well as an aid with regard to other aspects of drug development (i.e. approvals of clinical trials by Ethics Committees, selection of clinical trial endpoints and drug discovery targets, and interpretation of efficacy and safety results of clinical trials), and are discussed below.

Lilford and Jackson (1995) introduced the concept of 'equipoise', the condition which applies when there is no preference between the treatment options to be compared, within the context of conducting ethical randomization in clinical trials and the approval of such trials by Ethics Committees. Using probability estimates, 'effective equipoise' occurs when the most likely results of a proposed trial are thought to be an improvement sufficient, but only just sufficient, to compensate for the disadvantage of the treatment with the greatest 'costs'. These 'costs' are side effects when viewed from the point of view of the individual patient, or the combination of those side effects and monetary costs when viewed from the perspective of society.

Bjornsson (1997) developed a systematic classification for the categorization of therapeutic effects of individual medicines based on their relationships to the underlying disease processes being treated or prevented, rather than on the pharmacological or biochemical effects of the individual medicines. This matrix method is based on six categories of therapeutic specificities and three levels of therapeutic effectiveness.

Category 0 includes medicines or medicine uses that prevent the development of a disease when none exists; Category I, those that affect aetiological factors of a disease; Category II, those that affect specific disease processes; Category III, those that affect specific disease manifestations; Category IV, those that affect non-specific disease manifestations or symptoms; and Category V includes medicines used to diagnose or facilitate treatment of a disease. Level 1 of therapeutic effectiveness applies to medicines that involve excellent, major or maximum effectiveness; Level 2 applies to medicines that involve good, substantial or medium effectiveness; and Level 3 applies to medicines that involve poor, marginal or minimum effectiveness. By providing a framework for comparisons across different therapeutic agents, be it based on benefits but ignoring risks, this matrix evaluation method may have implications in choosing clinical trial endpoints and selecting drug discovery targets.

Shakespeare *et al.* (2001) presented a new concept for the calculation and interpretation of the efficacy and safety results of a clinical trial. As discussed further in Chapter 3, they proposed to use confidence intervals and plotting of clinical significance curves and risk-benefit contours.

Use of models by regulatory authorities

At the outset, it is important to note again that benefit–risk analysis undertaken by regulators is not based on a precise mathematical equation and is invariably judgemental, making the term 'benefit–risk ratio' a misnomer (Waller, 2001). Already in 1973, it was acknowledged that regulatory authorities were poorly equipped to undertake the sophisticated benefit–risk analyses, and that better methodology was required (Wardell, 1973). As will be shown below, this is still the case today, and no standardized method or model is available for regulatory authorities.

Only three models for benefit–risk assessment of medicines for use by regulatory authorities are described in the literature: (1) the 'Principle of Threes' grading system developed by Edwards *et al.* (1996), (2) the TURBO model developed by Amery (CIOMS Working Group IV, 1998), and (3) the Evidence-based Benefit and Risk Model developed by Beckmann (1999). The first two methods are also described in the Report of the CIOMS Working Group IV entitled 'Benefit/risk Balance for Marketed Drugs: Evaluating Safety Signals'. All three models have been developed either within the scope of the evaluation of the benefit–risk balance of marketed medicines because of a safety concern, and/or by people who are primarily involved in pharmacovigilance activities. The primary focus of these models is therefore more on safety than efficacy, and more on the re-evaluation of marketed medicines than the evaluation of new medicines.

Edwards set out to establish a simple and fast methodology to evaluate the benefit–risk balance of a medicine. He proposed a 'Principle of Threes' structure to evaluate the benefit–risk balance of medicines. The model is based upon the concepts of seriousness, duration and incidence, as related to disease indication, disease ameliora- tion by a medicine, and the adverse effects ascribed to the medicine. The TURBO model is a quantitative and graphical approach to benefit–risk analysis, developed by Amery. This method tries to quantify the benefits and risks of a medicine in a given indication, and both factors are then displayed on the TURBO diagram. Beckmann described a model in which the evidence-weighted benefit is balanced against the sum of all evidence weighted risks. All three models are reviewed in detail in Chapter 3. It is however important to note that none of these models have been well-accepted nor are they used in practice by regulatory authorities.

Meyboom and Egberts (1999) suggested that in an ideal situation, when extensive or even complete qualitative and quantitative data are available, it should be possible to calculate the positive and negative effects of a medicine, using quality-of-life assess- ment methodology. The cumulative risk of a medicine can be calculated as the Drug-Attributed Loss of Quality-Adjusted Life Years (DALQALY). Similarly, the benefit can be presented as Drug-Attributed Gain of Quality-Adjusted Life Years (DAGQALY). If benefit and risk are expressed in the same measure (standard unit), the net benefit of the medicine can be calculated by subtracting the risk from the total benefit. Otherwise an equation can be made (of risk units per unit of benefit). However, the collection of the body of evidence needed for such assessments requires large-scale, intensive and continuous data-gathering made into a routine in medical and pharma- ceutical practice, which is not a reality today. Nevertheless, quality-of-life measures such as SF-36 are increasingly used for measuring health outcomes in clinical research (Garratt et al., 2002).

It should be noted that regulatory authorities seem to increasingly advocate the use of 'numbers needed to treat' (NNT) in product labelling, and hence in regulatory deci- sions. NNT is defined as the reciprocal of the absolute risk reduction due to a given therapy and conveys the effort that must be expended on average to accomplish a single, tangible, and positive outcome in a patient (Mancini and Schulzer, 1999). A quantitative method for benefit–risk assessment based on an adjusted NNT approach has been reviewed (Holden, 2003). The concept and applicability of NNT will be discussed in detail in Chapter 3.

Another quantitative approach called minimum clinical efficacy (MCE) was first introduced by Djulbegovic et al. (1998) as a means of choosing high-dose or low-dose chemotherapy for the adjuvant treatment of breast cancer, and was fine-tuned for general use and applied by Holden et al. (2003a; 2003b). MCE of a new treatment is the minimal clinical efficacy needed for it to be worth considering as an alternative treatment after taking into account: (1) the efficacy of the standard treatment; (2) the adverse event profiles associated with the standard treatment and the new treatment; and (3) the risk of disease associated with no treatment. This method will be reviewed in Chapter 3.

In Japan, the use of the YUYOSEÏ instrument in clinical trials and hence in marketing authorization applications is mandatory. The YUYOSEÏ instrument is an assessment whereby each patient is considered as a whole with their safety and efficacy experience in a trial combined to obtain an overall outcome measure (Chuang-Stein, 1999). It is a global assessment given by the treating physician to reflect, in the physician's opinion, an individual's overall response to treatment. By its very definition, YUYOSEÏ has objective and subjective components, since the sense of well-being of a patient can be quite subjective. However, research has demonstrated that this utility evaluation system is unreliable because of poor intra-rater as well as inter-rater reproducibility (Naito, 1994).

In the absence of general standard models for benefit–risk assessment by regulatory authorities (except in Japan), it should also be noted that there are no such models for specific categories of medicines either. There is for example no standardized method of incorporating toxicity and tolerability information into decisions regarding the regulatory approval of new cancer treatments (Rothenberg et al., 2003). Hence there are no easy answers to questions such as whether a new agent that improves median survival time or time-to-tumour progression by a statistically significant 6-week margin be approved, even if it is associated with substantial rates of treatment-induced morbidity or mortality. Arlett suggested that for thrombolytic agents for the treatment of acute myocardial infarction, an estimate of the number of serious cases of haemorrhage per infarct prevented could be calculated when evaluating the balance of benefits and risks (Arlett, 2001). Methods for assessing the benefit–risk profile of oral triptans, vaccines and selective oestrogen receptor modulators are reviewed in Chapter 3.

Use of models by prescribers

It is recognized that prescribers need validated and interpreted data on the benefit–risk assessment of medicines, which should clearly define the benefit–risk relationship and put it in perspective with other therapeutic means. In addition, such data are required for ensuring that patients receive accurate and transparent information on the benefits and risks of medicines (Lehner et al., 2001). The intended use of benefit–risk assessments in the setting of clinical trials, be it individual clinical trials or all available clinical trials for a given medicine, is usually as a population-based assessment (Costantino, 2001). In contrast, in the clinical practice setting the intended use of benefit–risk assessment is as an individual patient-based assessment (Spilker 1994; Edwards and Hugman, 1997).

Costantino developed a tool for communicating to individual patients the results of the benefit–risk assessment of selective oestrogen receptor modulators (SERMs) like tamoxifen. He was of the opinion that without such a tool the communication of a benefit–risk assessment to an individual woman can be a difficult task because of the complicated interplay of numerous potential beneficial and detrimental effects of SERMs. The properties of an ideal tool were identified as a tool that: (1) avoids to the extent possible the use of probabilities or relative risks as these are entities that can be confusing to those not familiar with such statistical measures; (2) includes information on all potentially affected endpoints with consideration of effects grouped by the relative severity of the different endpoints; and (3) provides a presentation that summarizes the results of the benefit–risk assessment that is limited to one page. The approach to providing information in the tool is based on describing the effects of therapy in terms of the number of cases expected to occur over 5 years of follow-up among 10 000 women of the same race, age group, and predicted breast cancer risk as the individual being assessed. The tool provides a comparison of the number of cases expected if none of the 10 000 was treated with the number of cases that may be prevented or caused if all 10 000 women were treated. Although the methodology was specifically developed and applied to the use of tamoxifen, it is a generalized procedure that can be readily modified and applied to other forms of therapy including other SERMs.

Loke *et al.* (2003) developed a benefit–risk analysis of aspirin therapy which allowed quantifying the reduction in cardiovascular events and the increase in gastrointestinal haemorrhage in an individual patient, according to the individual risk profile. The absolute treatment effects were calculated from estimates of baseline risks for cardiovascular events and gastrointestinal haemorrhage, and relative risks of these events with treatment. Baseline cardiovascular risks were derived from existing risk scores, and baseline risk of gastrointestinal haemorrhage from an observational cohort study. Changes in relative risk were obtained from clinical trial data. The use of a graphical technique incorporating these baseline risks should enable doctors and patients to assess easily the benefit–risk ratio of aspirin in a particular individual.

Conclusions on the existing models

Based on this review of the literature, it is apparent that there are relatively few general methods and models for benefit–risk assessment, in particular for use by regulatory authorities. None of these methods seem to be widely accepted and applied. In general, there appears to be a lack of a methodological framework and guidance with regard to the relevant benefit and risk criteria to be considered for benefit–risk assessments, and with regard to trading-off the benefits and risks of medicines. Furthermore, there appears to be room for a better general, broadly applicable method for benefit–risk assessments of medicines.

1.9   DISCUSSIONS WITH STAKEHOLDERS ON THE CONCEPTS AND MODELS FOR BENEFIT–RISK EVALUATION

The above discussed framework, concepts and models for benefit–risk evaluations were extensively discussed with stakeholders, including representatives from the pharmaceutical industry and from health authorities, in two workshops organized by CMR International Institute for Regulatory Science. The conclusions of both workshops, which further elaborate on and illustrate the content of this chapter, are included in Appendix 1.

CHAPTER 2

Criteria for a Benefit–Risk Model: a Conceptual Framework

2.1 INTRODUCTION

A number of authors either working for regulatory authorities or in organizations involved in drug development recognize that the demonstration of a favourable benefit–risk profile of a medicine is a complex issue that needs to take into account numerous factors (Spilker, 1994; Arlett, 2001; Pignatti *et al.*, 2002). However, no single literature source exists which identifies and establishes all of these factors, which can be grouped according to a number of criteria that pertain to efficacy, a number of criteria that pertain to safety, and potentially a number of other criteria (for example the effectiveness of the medicine in the marketplace).

Hence, the purpose of this chapter is to conduct a detailed review of the benefit and risk criteria that are currently used or should be used for benefit–risk assessment of new medicines as well as marketed medicines. This review is based on a discussion of regulatory guidelines issued by regulatory authorities and on pertinent scientific literature. From this review, a list of benefit and risk criteria which ideally should be considered for benefit–risk assessment is proposed, and for each criterion a definition is provided as well as a rationale why that specific criterion should be taken into account for benefit–risk assessment. The validity of this list was checked by means of a questionnaire to experts in the field, who were asked to indicate if, in their view, each of these benefit and risk criteria should be taken into account for benefit–risk assessment.

The list of criteria established in this chapter is the benchmark against which existing models were reviewed (Chapter 3), and it was used as the basis to develop a new model

Benefit-Risk Appraisal of Medicines   Filip Mussen, Sam Salek, Stuart Walker
© 2009 John Wiley & Sons, Ltd

(Chapter 5). As part of the development of this new model, each criterion that was identified and justified in this chapter was further validated.

2.2   REGULATORY GUIDELINES ON BENEFIT AND RISK CRITERIA

The focus of this research will be on the benefit–risk assessment of medicines within the scope of the registration of new medicines and the re-evaluation of marketed medicines. Both these processes are essentially driven by specific regulations and guidelines issued by the regulatory authorities. The health authorities, such as the European Medicines Evaluation Agency in the EU and the FDA in the United States, are responsible for conducting these benefit–risk assessments in accordance with the regulations, and primarily based on the data provided by the pharmaceutical companies. Hence it is essential to consider these regulations as the framework into which any model for benefit–risk assessment has to fit. In addition, the regulations and the more detailed guidelines define the scope and essential characteristics of a model, because they establish the efficacy and safety data that must be generated for each medicine. The regulations and guidelines that will be taken into account in the next chapters for the review of the existing models and the construction of a new model are those applicable in the European Union, and those in force in the United States. The reason for focusing on the EU and the US regulations is that these are the two largest pharmaceutical markets in the world. The Japanese requirements will also be considered to a certain extent, as discussed below.

A very important part of the regulations and guidelines on medicines in the EU and United States are the ICH guidelines. The International Conference on Harmonisation of Technical Requirements for Registration of Pharmaceuticals for Human Use (ICH) is a project which started in 1991 that brings together the regulatory authorities of Europe, Japan and the United States, and experts from the pharmaceutical industry in the three regions to achieve greater harmonization in the interpretation and application of technical guidelines and requirements for product registration. The goal of this harmonization is to reduce or obviate the need to duplicate the testing carried out during the research and development of new medicines (ICH, 2004). The overall objective of such harmonization is the more economical use of human, animal and material resources, and the elimination of unnecessary delays in the global development and availability of new medicines whilst maintaining safeguards on quality, safety and efficacy, and regulatory obligations to protect public health. By 2008, ICH had issued 23 guidelines on 'quality' topics (i.e. those relating to chemical and pharmaceutical quality assurance), 16 guidelines on 'safety' topics (i.e. those relating to *in vitro* and *in vivo* preclinical studies), 20 'efficacy' topics (i.e. those relating to clinical studies and pharmacovigilance activities), and 8 multidisciplinary topics. Most of these guidelines have been implemented in the three ICH regions, and are also used as a reference in other countries (e.g. Canada). Therefore, wherever in the next chapters the applicable regulations will be reviewed for the evaluation of the current models for benefit–risk assessment and for the construction of a new model, the ICH guidelines will be used as the primary reference. The establishment of the Global Cooperation Group has now allowed other regional regulatory authorities such as Asia Pacific Economic Cooperation (APEC), Association of Southeast Asian Nations (ASEAN), Gulf Cooperation Council (GCC), and Pan-American Network for Drug Regulation Harmonization (PANDRH) to participate (2005) and more recently (2008–2009) a number of Drug Regulatory Authorities from India, China, Russia, Brazil, Korea, Australia, Republic of China (Taiwan) and Singapore to contribute as well.

Two kinds of regulatory guidelines exist which discuss how benefit–risk assessment should be performed and what criteria should be considered: guidelines for the pharmaceutical industry on how benefit–risk should be described in the dossiers submitted to regulatory authorities, and internal guidelines for regulators which establish how they should describe benefit and risk in their assessment reports and conclusions. As will be shown in this section, few of these guidelines identify comprehensively and fully the relevant benefit and risk criteria that should be taken into account.

The most comprehensive list of relevant benefit and risk criteria can probably be found in the ICH guideline on the Common Technical Document which defines the presentation and content of the marketing authorization dossier in the United States, EU and Japan (ICH, 2000). In particular, the guideline describes in detail which criteria should be discussed in the 'Overview of Efficacy', 'Overview of Safety', and 'Benefits and Risks Conclusions' of the Clinical Overview (Module 2.5), which is intended to provide a critical analysis of the clinical data in the Common Technical document. In the EU, a CHMP guideline exists on the content of the day 80 assessment report for new applications in the centralized procedure (which implicitly also covers the scope of the actual assessment). This guideline describes how the clinical experience should be discussed as well as what questions should be addressed in the clinical conclusions. The 2004 version of this guideline was used for populating Table 2.1, although the latest version was issued in 2006 (European Medicines Agency, 2004). In the United States, no such guidance exists to date but a template for the clinical review, which is issued as part of the medical review, was published in 2004 based on an earlier template from the Oncology Division (FDA, 2004). Table 2.1 lists which criteria are included in each of these three documents.

As can be noted from Table 2.1, there are significant differences between the three documents in terms of the listed efficacy and safety criteria. Also, some criteria are actually a grouping of different criteria (e.g. safety criterion no. 12 – reactions due to overdose; the potential for dependence, rebound phenomena and abuse, or lack of data on these issues), or are very broad, not well-defined criteria which overlap with other criteria (e.g. safety criterion no. 20 – adverse events). Therefore, in the next section a systematic review will be conducted to identify and define the relevant criteria based on the above list and based on additional literature references.

Table 2.1   The benefit and risk criteria required to be covered in the Common Technical Document ('ICH'), in the EU assessment reports ('EU'), and in US Medical Reviews ('FDA')

	ICH	EU	FDA
Efficacy[a]			
1. Relevant features of the patient populations, including demographic features, disease stage and other potential important covariates, any important patient populations excluded from critical studies, participation of children and elderly and the population that would be expected to receive the medicine after marketing	√	√	√
2. Implications of the study designs, including selection of patients, duration of studies and choice of endpoints and control groups	√	√	√
3. For non-inferiority trials used to demonstrate efficacy, the evidence supporting a determination that the trial had assay sensitivity and justifying the choice of the non-inferiority margin	√		
4. Statistical methods and any issues that could affect the interpretation of the study results	√	√	√
5. Similarities and differences in results among studies, or in different patient subgroups within studies, and their effect upon the interpretation of the efficacy data	√		√
6. Observed relationships between efficacy, dose and dosage regimen for each indication, in both the overall population and in the different patient subgroups	√	√	√
7. Support for the applicability to a specific region of data generated in another region	√		
8. For a medicine intended for long-term use, efficacy findings pertinent to the maintenance of long-term efficacy and the establishment of long-term dosage	√	√	
9. Data suggesting that treatment results can be improved through plasma concentration monitoring, if any, and documentation for an optimal plasma concentration range	√		
10. The clinical relevance of the magnitude of the observed effects	√	√	√
11. If surrogate endpoints are relied upon, the nature and magnitude of expected clinical benefit and the basis for these expectations	√	√	√
12. Efficacy in special populations	√	√	
13. Statistical evaluation of the results		√	√
14. Supportive studies		√	
Safety[a]			
1. Adverse effects characteristic of the pharmacological class	√		√
2. Special approaches to monitoring for particular adverse events	√		√[b]
3. Relevant animal toxicology and product quality information	√	√	√
4. The nature of the patient population and the extent of exposure	√		√

5. Common and non-serious adverse events	√		√
6. Serious adverse events	√	√	√
7. Similarities and differences in results among studies, and their effect upon the interpretation of the safety data	√		
8. Any differences in rate of adverse events in population subgroups	√	√	√
9. Relation of adverse effects to dose, dose regimen and treatment duration	√	√	√
10. Long-term safety	√	√	
11. Methods to prevent, mitigate or manage adverse events	√		
12. Reactions due to overdose; the potential for dependence, rebound phenomena and abuse, or lack of data on these issues	√		√
13. World-wide marketing experience	√		
14. Support for the applicability to a region of data generated in another region	√		
15. Any risks to the patient of known and potential interactions, including food–drug and drug–drug interactions	√	√	√
16. Any potential effect of the medicine that might affect the ability to drive or operate heavy machinery	√		
17. Deaths		√	√
18. Incidence of adverse drug reactions			√
19. Human reproduction data			√
20. Adverse events		√	
21. Laboratory findings, vital signs, ECGs		√	√
22. Discontinuation due to adverse events		√	√

[a]In the first column of the table, the wording used in the ICH Common Technical Document was used for each criterion that was covered in this ICH document, since that guideline applies to both the EU and US, in contrast to the other two guidelines.
[b]The FDA Clinical Review template covers specifically immunogenicity (for monoclonal antibodies), the effect on growth (for medicines for children), human carcinogenicity (for medicines for chronic use), and QTc prolongation.
ECG, electrocardiogram.

2.3   IDENTIFICATION, DEFINITION AND RATIONALE OF RELEVANT BENEFIT AND RISK CRITERIA

Prerequisites

The above mentioned guidelines as well as other sources (Spilker, 1994; Beckmann, 1999) recognize that a separate benefit–risk assessment should be conducted for each indication, because medicines are clinically tested for each indication separately. In addition, it can be argued that the actual indication text as established in the product label should be the basis for defining the benefits and risks, as suggested in the US legislation which requires that a medicine is safe and effective under the conditions prescribed, recommended or suggested in the labelling (Federal Food, Drug and Cosmetic Act, 1997). As shown in the example which follows, the benefit–risk balance for an indication restricted to a specific subpopulation of people having the disease for which the medicine is developed is potentially different than for a broad indication for the whole population having the disease, because the evidence for efficacy and/or safety might be different in the restricted versus the broad population. Rosiglitazone is indicated in the United States both as first-line monotherapy and as combination therapy in patients with type 2 diabetes mellitus (Physician's Desk Reference, 2008), whilst in the EU the indication is restricted to second-line combination treatment in patients with insufficient glycaemic control (CHMP, 2008). The proof of efficacy and/or safety and thus the benefit–risk balance might be different for monotherapy and a broad combination therapy indication (United States) versus a second-line combination therapy indication (EU). Actually, the EU regulators had restricted the indication because in their view the benefit–risk balance of the broader US indication was not positive (CHMP, 2008).

Similarly, selecting the dose range consists of establishing dosage limits that provide an acceptable benefit–risk ratio (Cocchetto and Nardi, 1986). Inversely, a benefit–risk profile for a given medicine is specific for a given indication and for a given dose or dose range for that indication as defined in the product label. Establishing a lower dose might reduce efficacy and/or dose-related side effects, whilst establishing a higher dose might increase efficacy and/or dose-related side effects, both of which can influence the benefit–risk profile.

Lastly, it can also be argued that the benefit–risk profile is partly determined by the contraindications of a medicine as established in the product label. Theoretically, if a medicine is 'unsafe' in a specific patient population (which has a negative impact on the risk profile), the benefit–risk profile for the populations targeted in the label can be improved by contraindicating the use of the medicine in that patient population. This concept of determining the risk profile within the context of the product label is suggested in the US legislation, which requires that a medicine is safe under the conditions prescribed, recommended or suggested in the labelling. Although this concept is not discussed in the literature, it has been endorsed during a number of presentations that were given on benefit–risk assessment (Mussen, 2001, 2002).

Overall, there are thus three prerequisites for benefit–risk assessment, which define the scope of the assessment: (1) the indication; (2) the dosage for that particular indication; and (3) the contraindications, as established in the product label.

Benefit criteria

Identification of the relevant clinical trials

Before establishing the relevant benefit criteria related to the evidence of efficacy of medicines, it is necessary to determine which clinical trials should be taken into account for this purpose. In a marketing authorization application for a new medicine, a significant number of phase I, phase II and phase III clinical trials are reported and are assessed by the regulatory authorities. Subsequently, a number of additional trials are usually carried out, some of which might be of importance for a post-approval re-assessment of the benefit–risk profile of the medicine. Hence the clinical trials on which the efficacy criteria should be applied must be defined at the outset, and it should be ensured that those trials are relevant to the claimed indication and dosage, as discussed in the previous section.

The ICH note for guidance on general considerations for clinical trials (1997) includes a robust methodology for this purpose. It classifies clinical studies according to objectives as follows:

- human pharmacology (to assess tolerance, define/describe pharmacokinetics and pharmacodynamics, explore drug metabolism and drug interactions, estimate activity);

- therapeutic exploratory (to explore use for the targeted indication, estimate dosage for subsequent studies, provide basis for confirmatory study design, endpoints, methodologies);

- therapeutic confirmatory (to demonstrate/confirm efficacy, establish safety profile, provide an adequate basis for assessing the benefit/risk relationship to support licensing, establish dose-response relationship);

- therapeutic use (to refine understanding of benefit/risk relationship in general or special populations and/or environments, identify less common adverse reactions, refine dosing recommendation).

The phase III programme, which is intended to provide an adequate basis for marketing approval, usually consists of therapeutic confirmatory studies (ICH, 1997). Hence, the relevant clinical trials for determining the efficacy of a new medicine are usually the 'therapeutic confirmatory' studies. The relevant clinical trials for determining the efficacy of a marketed medicine might include, in addition to therapeutic confirmatory studies, also phase IV studies which begin after the initial approval of the medicine and which usually consist of 'therapeutic use' trials. Phase IV studies of particular interest in this respect are studies to support use under the approved indication, such as morbidity/mortality studies that might provide a new perspective on the benefit of a medicine.

In conclusion, the therapeutic confirmatory studies and therapeutic use studies (if available) that are relevant to the claimed indication and dosage should be identified, and the appropriate benefit criteria, which will be discussed in the next section, should be applied on each of those studies. For the purpose of this chapter, those studies will be called 'pivotal studies'.

Efficacy versus comparator and its clinical relevance

This criterion pertains to the evidence of efficacy (magnitude of the treatment effect) and its clinical relevance from clinical trials is mentioned in the ICH, EU and FDA documents (Table 2.1 – Efficacy criterion no. 10 – the clinical relevance of the magnitude of the observed effects) and should be applied to each pivotal trial. It is clearly the most important criterion with regard to benefit as it represents the overall benefit of the medicine. Two questions should be addressed in this respect: (1) which efficacy variables from the pivotal trials should be taken into account, and (2) how can clinical relevance be determined. The complexity of these issues and of benefit assessment in general was recently reviewed by Califf (2007).

The ICH guideline on statistical principles for clinical trials (1998) addresses the issue of efficacy variables. As per this guideline, the primary variable (primary end-point) should be the variable capable of providing the most clinically relevant and convincing evidence directly related to the primary objective of the trial. There should generally be only one primary variable, which is usually an efficacy variable because the primary objective of most confirmatory trials is to provide strong scientific evidence regarding efficacy. Sometimes the primary variable is a composite variable which combines multiple measurements associated with the primary objective of the trial. The primary variable is generally used to estimate the sample size of the trial. Secondary variables are either supportive measurements related to the primary objective or measurements of effects related to secondary objectives. Thus, for the efficacy demonstrated with a medicine in a given trial and its clinical relevance, the results with regard to the primary efficacy variable should be taken into account, because the primary variable provides the clinically most relevant evidence for efficacy. As will be discussed in the next section, results with regard to secondary objectives can be considered as supportive and should be taken into account separately.

Determining the clinical relevance of the efficacy is essentially a judgement call (Fitzgerald, 1987), and in Chapter 5 a specific methodology will be proposed for this purpose. Nevertheless, it is important to describe in this section the benchmark against which this judgement call will be made, which depends on the design of the pivotal trials. The most common clinical trial design for confirmatory trials is the parallel group design in which subjects are randomized to one of two or more arms, each arm being allocated a different treatment (ICH, 1998). As stated by the ICH, scientifically, efficacy is most convincingly established by demonstrating superiority to placebo in a placebo-controlled trial (which is not always possible ethically), or showing superiority to an active control treatment (these are called 'superiority' trials). However, in some cases a new medicine is compared to an active reference treatment without the objective of showing superiority, either in an 'equivalence' trial (a trial with the primary objective of showing that the response to two or more treatments differs by an amount which is clinically unimportant), or in a 'non-inferiority' trial (a trial with the primary objective of showing that the response to the investigational product is not clinically inferior to a comparative agent). Active control equivalence or non-inferiority trials may also incorporate a placebo, and pursue multiple goals in one trial by also establishing superiority to placebo and hence validate the trial design. Thus, if a pivotal trial was a superiority trial versus placebo, the clinical relevance of the efficacy of the medicine with respect to the primary variable will have to be considered against the placebo. In contrast, if one or more of the pivotal trials were superiority, equivalence or non-inferiority trials versus an active control, the clinical relevance of the efficacy with respect to the primary variable will be considered against the active treatment. Thus by definition such trials will allow for a judgement of the relative benefit of the new medicine versus the active comparator. In this respect it is very important that the active comparator is a widely used therapy whose efficacy in the relevant indication has been clearly established and quantified in well-designed and well-documented superiority trials and which can be reliably expected to exhibit similar efficacy in the contemplated active control trial (ICH, 1998).

Other efficacy criteria to be applied on each pivotal study

There are a number of other specificities or data related to the design, conduct and results of a pivotal study which could either confirm the efficacy and its clinical relevance as discussed in the previous section, or (partly) invalidate it. As such they can have an impact on the benefit–risk balance because they can negatively influence the benefit of a medicine. A number of the efficacy criteria listed in Table 2.1 pertain to these trial specificities and data: criteria nos. 1, 2, 3, 4, 5, 8, 11, 12 and 13. Whilst this list of criteria was used as a basis, it was felt that the criteria should be better defined and that if possible a shorter list should be established, also based on a review of the scientific literature. Therefore, a list of six criteria was established, of which the first three (i.e. 'design, conduct and statistical adequacy of the trial', 'clinical relevance of the primary endpoints', and 'representativeness of the studied population for the population targeted in the label') pertain to study design/conduct, and the last three (i.e. 'statistical significance of the efficacy results', 'evidence for the efficacy in relevant subgroups', and 'efficacy as per the results of non-primary endpoints') to study results.

'Design, conduct and statistical adequacy of the trial'

For each trial, the question should be asked whether the results represent an unbiased estimate of the treatment effect, or whether they were influenced in some systematic fashion to lead to a false conclusion? This question has to do with the validity and accuracy of the results and considers whether the reported treatment effect represents the true direction and magnitude of the treatment effect (Guyatt *et al.*, 1993).

Guyatt *et al.* suggested that the following key questions should be addressed with regard to the validity of the results of a trial: was the assignment of patients to treatment randomized? Were all patients who entered the trial properly accounted for and attributed at its conclusion? Were patients, their clinicians and study personnel 'blind' to treatment? Were the groups similar at the start of the trial? Aside from the experimental intervention, were the groups treated equally? The ICH guideline on general considerations for clinical trials (1997) also lists a number of considerations with regard to the design, conduct and analysis of a trial. These considerations pertain to: (1) the selection of subjects (the stage of development and the indication to be studied should be taken into account in selecting the subject population, as should prior non-clinical and clinical knowledge); (2) the selection of the control group (comparisons may be made with placebo, no treatment, active controls or of different doses of the medicine under investigation); (3) the number of subjects (the size of the trial is influenced by the disease to be investigated, the objective of the study and the study endpoints); (4) the response variables (should be defined prospectively, giving descriptions of methods of observation and quantification); (5) the methods to minimize or assess bias (methods for randomization, blinding and compliance); (6) the conduct of a trial (should be conducted according to Good Clinical Practice); and (7) the analysis of the trial (should be done according to the analysis plan). Although it is not the purpose to describe in this section in detail all above mentioned prerequisites for producing valid and accurate clinical trial results, a few issues warrant further explanation.

- Since it is essential to avoid or minimize bias in clinical trials, it is worth noting that Greenhalgh (1997) described the particular sources of systematic bias in randomized controlled trials, which are selection bias (systematic differences in the comparison groups attributable to incomplete randomization), performance bias (systematic differences in the care provided apart from the intervention being evaluated), exclusion bias (systematic differences in withdrawals from the trial), and detection bias (systematic differences in outcome assessment).

- The conduct of a trial should be in accordance with the principles of Good Clinical Practice, which is an international ethical and scientific quality standard for designing, conducting, recording and reporting trials that involve the participation of human subjects (ICH, 1996). Compliance with this standard provides assurance that, amongst other things, the clinical trial data are credible. The principles of ICH which pertain to the quality of a trial are that: (1) clinical trials should be scientifically sound, and described in a clear, detailed protocol; (2) a trial should be conducted in compliance with the protocol that has received prior ethics committee approval; (3) each individual involved in conducting a trial should be qualified by education, training, and experience to perform his or her respective tasks; (4) all clinical trial information should be recorded, handled and stored in a way that allows its accurate reporting, interpretation and verification; (5) investigational products should be manufactured, handled and stored in accordance with applicable good manufacturing practice, and used in accordance with the approved protocol; and (6) systems with procedures that assure the quality of every aspect of the trial should be implemented.

- It is essential that statistical principles are adhered to for each trial, and that a sound statistical methodology is used in order to minimize bias and maximize precision. These principles are established in the ICH guideline on statistical principles for clinical trials (1998) and are also described in many textbooks. It is therefore not the purpose to provide more details on these principles in this section.

In conclusion, the criterion 'design, conduct and statistical adequacy of the trial' is a broad criterion which encompasses potential issues with regard to the design and conduct of a clinical trial including the statistical methodology used in the trial. The reason for establishing this as a criterion to be applied on each pivotal study is that it assesses a key question which is whether the results represent an unbiased and accurate estimate of the treatment effect observed in the study.

'Clinical relevance of the primary endpoints'

The primary endpoint(s) should be the variable capable of providing the most clinically relevant and convincing evidence directly related to the primary objective of the study (ICH, 1998). The selection of the primary variable should reflect the accepted norms and standards in the relevant field of research. The use of a reliable and validated variable with which experience has been gained either in earlier studies or in published literature is recommended. There should be sufficient evidence that the primary variable can provide a valid and reliable measure of some clinically relevant and important treatment benefit in the patient population described by the inclusion and exclusion criteria. In many cases however, the approach of assessing subject outcome may not be straightforward (ICH, 1998). Hence it is considered appropriate for each primary endpoint to establish a separate criterion with regard to the clinical relevance of the primary endpoint.

For medicines for which the effect can be measured in terms of the incidence of mortality, there is clearly no issue, but for many trials surrogate endpoints or measurements of symptomatic (e.g. pain), functional (e.g. mobility), psychological (e.g. anxiety) or social (e.g. inconvenience) will have to be used and such endpoints are fraught with problems (Greenhalgh, 1997). A surrogate endpoint is a variable that provides an indirect measurement of effect in situations where direct measurement of clinical effect is not feasible or practical (ICH, 1998). The approval of a medicine on the basis of its impact on a surrogate endpoint is not new. For years medicines have been marketed based on their ability to lower blood pressure, without data on their ability to prevent heart attacks, strokes, etc. (Lasagna, 1998).

To illustrate that the clinical relevance and treatment benefit of the primary variable are not always clear-cut, the following examples of primary variables agreed upon by the CHMP (formerly the Committee for Medicinal Products, CPMP) in a number of different disease areas are provided.

- For symptom-modifying medicines for the treatment of osteoarthritis, two primary endpoints are recommended: pain as measured by self-assessment with a validated method such as visual analogue or Likert scales, and functional disability as measured with a disease-specific and joint-specific instrument such as the Western Ontario and MacMaster Universities (WOMAC) index or the Lequesne index (Committee for Medicinal Products, 1998).

- For medicines for the treatment of Alzheimer's disease (AD), several variables may be used because: (1) there is no single test that encompasses the broad range of heterogeneous manifestations of dementia in AD; (2) there is no ideal measurement instrument at present; and (3) demented patients are poor observers and reporters of their own symptoms and behaviour, and therefore evaluations by relatives or nurses should be part of the assessment but this could cause bias (CPMP, 1997a). In the absence of a single well-accepted variable, it is required to specify as primary endpoints a cognitive measurement (such as the Alzheimer's Disease Assessment Scale (ADAS) cognitive subscale), a functional measurement (such as an Activities of Daily Living assessment), and a global measurement.

- For anticancer medicines, appropriate primary endpoints for confirmatory studies include progression-free/recurrence-free/relapse-free survival, overall survival, response rate, and symptom control/quality of life (CPMP, 2003a). In addition, the guideline stipulates that the selected primary endpoint should be based on clinical relevance and methodological considerations and that the study should be designed accordingly.

- For medicines to treat lipid disorders, the primary endpoint in confirmatory clinical trials to support an indication for primary hypercholesterolaemia is reduction in low-density lipoprotein (LDL)-cholesterol, which is a surrogate endpoint (CPMP, 2003c). Demonstration of a reduction in terms of morbidity and mortality is not required because of the direct correlation between LDL-cholesterol-lowering and improved morbidity and mortality (which has been demonstrated in epidemiological studies) and on the condition that from the clinical program there is no suspicion of a detrimental effect on both cardiovascular and non-cardiovascular morbidity and mortality.

In conclusion, in a number of disease areas, confirmatory trials use primary endpoints of which the clinical relevance is not necessarily fully established, either because surrogate endpoints are used or because there is no ideal endpoint that has been identified. Therefore, it is appropriate to establish a specific efficacy criterion which assesses the clinical relevance of the primary endpoint(s).

'Representativeness of the studied population for the population targeted in the label'

The nature of pivotal clinical trials makes it difficult to evaluate the benefits of medicines for the universe of potential users as established in the label. Most pivotal trials have increasingly lengthy lists of inclusion and exclusion criteria (Lasagna, 1998). The trial patients are usually not receiving any other medicine and are usually not suffering from more than one disease, and this approach is scientifically clean, but makes it difficult to guide practice in relation to wider patient groups (Greenhalgh, 1997). In addition, a randomised controlled trial may for example be restricted to patients with moderate to severe forms of a disease such as heart failure, a policy that could lead to false conclusions about the treatment of mild heart failure. The ICH guideline on statistical principles for clinical trials recognizes that in the earlier phases of drug development the choice of subjects for a clinical trial may be heavily influenced by the wish to maximize the chance of observing specific clinical effects of interest, and hence they may come from a very narrow subgroup of the total patient population for which the drug may eventually be indicated (ICH, 1998). However, in confirmatory trials the subjects should more closely mirror the target population and it is therefore in these trials generally helpful to relax the inclusion and exclusion criteria as much as possible within the target population, while maintaining sufficient homogeneity to permit precise estimation of treatment effects. No individual clinical trial can be expected to be totally representative of future users (ICH, 1998), and therefore it is considered appropriate to establish a specific efficacy criterion which pertains to the representativeness of the studied population in relation to the population targeted in the label. The above ICH guideline refers to this as 'generalizability' or 'generalization' and defines this as the extent to which the findings of a clinical trial can be reliably extrapolated from the subjects who participated in the trial to a broader patient population and a broader range of clinical settings.

'Statistical significance of the efficacy results'

The statistical section of the protocol of a clinical trial should specify the hypotheses that are to be tested and/or the treatment effects which are to be estimated in order to satisfy the primary objectives of the trial (ICH, 1998). Significance testing usually quantifies the strength of evidence in terms of probabilities (p-values) to reject the null hypothesis of no treatment effect (Pocock, 1996), the conventional level of statistical significance being a p-value of 0.05 (FDA, 1998). The estimates of treatment effect should be accompanied by confidence intervals, whenever possible (ICH, 1998). Whilst in simple terms the results of a trial with regard to the primary variable(s) are either statistically significant ($p \leq 0.05$) or not statistically significant (in which case the trial should be discounted as a therapeutic confirmatory trial because the result would be a false positive), there is a case to be made for the p-value to be judged using a more subtle approach, as illustrated by the following two opposite examples.

- The FDA considers a statistically very persuasive finding to be one of the require-ments for a single adequate and well-controlled study to be sufficient for supporting an effectiveness claim (FDA, 1998). A statistically very persuasive finding is further defined by the FDA as a very low p-value (thus presumably much lower than 0.05).

- Pocock argues that the choice of the level of the p-value (for example 0.05) is arbitrary and that it must be recognized that there is precious little difference between $p = 0.06$ and $p = 0.04$ (Pocock, 1996). This implies that even a study with a p-value of 0.06 should perhaps not be entirely discounted, since a two-tailed p-value of 0.06 means an error rate in the efficacy (false positive) tail of 0.03 or only one in approximately 33. In general a lower p-value is obtained if more patients were included in the study. A similar reasoning can be made for the 95 % confidence interval.

Thus, it is valuable to establish statistical significance as a separate efficacy criterion so that the level of statistical significance can be taken into account for the overall value of a given pivotal clinical trial, with a p-value which is borderline too high still getting some credit and a p-value which is well below the predefined level getting more credit than a p-value just below the required level.

'Evidence for the efficacy in relevant subgroups'

The treatment effect may vary with subgroup, for example the effect may decrease with age or may be larger in a particular diagnostic category of patients. In some cases such interactions are anticipated or are of particular interest (e.g. in the elderly) and hence a subgroup analysis or a statistical model including interactions is part of the statistical analysis. In other cases subgroup or interaction analyses are exploratory (ICH, 1998). Subgroup analysis should in principle be performed for each randomized clinical trial (Moher et al., 2001). For example, in the Studies of Left Ventricular Dysfunction (SOLVD) trial the effects were generally consistent among patients in New York Heart Association (NYHA) functional class I, II and III, but in patients in NYHA class IV there was no difference between enalapril and placebo in terms of mortality (The SOLVD Investigators, 1991). Such a decreased/absent effect in a particular subgroup may be relevant for the overall benefit of a medicine (as might be an increased effect) and should therefore be specifically assessed for most medicines depending on their nature and indications.

'Efficacy as per the results of the non-primary endpoints'

Secondary endpoints are either supportive measurements related to the primary objec-tive, or measurements of effects related to secondary objectives (ICH, 1998). The sample size and the power of a trial are usually not based on secondary variables, which is another reason why these results should be considered as supportive efficacy information. Nevertheless, secondary endpoints usually provide additional efficacy information and are required by regulatory authorities for trials in a number of fields.

For example, this suggests the following secondary endpoints for new medicines for the treatment of heart failure: quality of life, exercise capacity, haemodynamic state, neuro-endocrine status, and physical signs and renal function (CPMP, 1999). Thus, results from secondary variables are important and supplement the results based on the primary endpoints, and therefore warrant a separate efficacy criterion.

Other general efficacy criteria

In addition to the benefit criteria which were established in the previous section for each pivotal trial, three general criteria were considered to be required to determine the full benefit picture of a medicine. These criteria pertain to the efficacy results from additional clinical trials ('efficacy as per the results of the relevant non-pivotal trials and extensions'), the effectiveness of medicines in practice ('anticipated patient compliance in market use'), and the degree of consistency of the results of the pivotal trials ('clustering [consistency] of results of the pivotal trials').

'Efficacy as per the results of the relevant non-pivotal trials and extensions'

Earlier in this chapter 'pivotal trials' were defined as therapeutic confirmatory studies (usually the phase III studies) and selected therapeutic use studies (if available) that are relevant to the claimed indication and dosage. A number of criteria were established, which essentially focused on determining the value of each trial with regard to establishing the efficacy (benefit) of the medicine in question. In addition to these trials, the results of a number of other trials might be available which can be considered to provide supportive information on the efficacy of a medicine (ICH, 1997). Examples of such trials are:

- some therapeutic exploratory trials such as early trials of relative short duration in well-defined narrow patient populations, and dose–response exploration studies

- some therapeutic use studies such as studies of additional endpoints, large simple trials and pharmacoeconomic studies

- some therapeutic confirmatory trials that are not phase III trials, such as dose–response studies, which serve for establishing the dose(s) for the phase III trials

- extensions of pivotal trials – although no definition was found in the literature or in regulatory guidelines of 'extension trials', such trials are continuations of the base trial with the objective to obtain longer term efficacy and safety information, under a new protocol and usually with a control group (in three-arm base trials with an active comparator and placebo, placebo patients are sometimes re-randomised to the experimental medicine or the active comparator).

Thus, the efficacy results of such trials provide additional supportive information on the efficacy of a medicine and should therefore be taken into account for establishing the benefit of a medicine. Although the concept of the assessment of all relevant efficacy information by distinguishing between pivotal data and supportive data is only captured in the EU guidance (criterion no. 14 in Table 2.1), it is considered to be the most efficient way to examine the efficacy of a product, in particular for marketed medicines for which there may be a wealth of clinical data available.

'Anticipated patient compliance in market use'

The report of World Health Organization on adherence of long-term therapies claims that in developed countries adherence among patients suffering from chronic diseases averages only 50%, and that the magnitude and impact of poor adherence in developing countries is assumed to be even higher (World Health Organization, 2003). Adherence was defined as:

> the extent to which a person's behaviour – taking medication, following a diet, and/or executing lifestyle changes, corresponds with agreed recommendations from a health care provider.

Thus, adherence was considered to be broader than patient compliance with medication. The report states that there is strong evidence that many patients with chronic illnesses such as asthma, hypertension and diabetes have difficulty adhering to their recommended regimens, and that this is the primary reason for suboptimal clinical benefit. For example, studies have shown that in many countries less than 25% of patients treated for hypertension achieve optimal blood pressure, and that the best available estimate is that poor adherence to therapy contributes to lack of good blood pressure control in more than two-thirds of people living with hypertension.

Clearly, adherence to therapy is a major issue which has not been fully addressed yet (Urquhart, 2001). It is known from multiple studies with a number of chronic medications that the greater the number of daily intakes of a medicine, the worse the compliance (Kruse *et al.*, 1991; Penfornis, 2003). In general, the longer the duration of therapy, the more frequent the dosing, and the more complex the regimen (e.g. multiple devices or tasks), the poorer the adherence of the patient (WHO, 2003). The WHO report reviews data which show that the complexity of the regimen including multiple daily dosing is an issue with regard to adherence in the treatment of asthma, cancer, depression, diabetes, epilepsy, HIV/AIDS and hypertension.

Thus, if two medicines for a given chronic treatment would have exactly the same efficacy and one would have a twice-a-day regimen and the other a once-a-day regimen, the effectiveness and thus the overall benefit of the latter would in theory be greater because of better patient compliance. Since the above data demonstrate that adherence to treatment is a major public health issue (although not mentioned in the benefit criteria in Table 2.1), a specific benefit criterion on patient compliance is warranted so that medicines which promote good adherence to therapy (simple regimen, easy administration) can get credit for these features.

'Clustering (consistency) of results of the pivotal trials'

Efficacy criterion no. 5 in Table 2.1, which is derived from the ICH Common Technical Document and the FDA Medical Review, encompasses the examination of similarities and differences in results among studies, and their effect upon the interpretation of the efficacy data. In the US, the FDA requires at least two adequate and well-controlled studies, each convincing on its own, to establish effectiveness (FDA, 1998). In the EU, similar requirements usually apply although they are not documented. The reasons for this FDA requirement are that: (1) any clinical trial may be subject to unanticipated, undetected, systematic biases, which may lead to flawed conclusions; (2) the inherent variability in biological systems may produce a positive trial result by chance alone; (3) results obtained in a single centre may be dependent on site or investigator specific factors; and (4) rarely, favourable efficacy results are the product of scientific fraud. Thus, independent substantiation of experimental results addresses such problems by providing consistency across more than one study, thus greatly reducing the possibility that a biased, chance, site-specific or fraudulent result will lead to an erroneous conclusion that a medicine is effective. The need for independent substantiation has often been referred to as the need for replication of the finding, which may not be the best term as it may imply that precise repetition of the same experiment in other patients by other investigators is the only means to substantiate a conclusion. According to the FDA, precise replication of a trial is only one of a number of possible means of obtaining independent substantiation of a clinical finding and, at times, can be less than optimal as it could leave the conclusions vulnerable to any systematic biases inherent to the particular study design. Results that are obtained from studies that are of different design and independent in execution may provide support for a conclusion of effectiveness that is as convincing as, or more convincing than, a repetition of the same study. Irrespective of the fact whether the pivotal studies are identical in design, the more consistency there is between the results of the pivotal trials, the more evidence there is for the effectiveness for a drug. This correlation justifies a specific criterion which has an impact on the benefit of a medicine.

Dismissed benefit (efficacy) criteria

The following three efficacy criteria listed in Table 2.1 were dismissed because they do not have a specific impact on the benefit of a medicine within the scope of the prerequisites defined earlier in this chapter.

- Efficacy criterion no. 6 – 'observed relationships between efficacy, dose and dosage regimen for each indication'. The specific reason for not taking into account this criterion is that the dosage, as established in the product label, is defined upfront and that all efficacy criteria are applied to the medicine with regard to that specific dosage.

- Efficacy criterion no. 7 – 'support for the applicability to a specific region of data generated in another region'. This is an ICH criterion which is of particular significance in Japan (which is one of the three ICH regions), since most medicines are first developed and filed for registration in Europe and the United States.

- Efficacy criterion no. 9 – 'data suggesting that treatment results can be improved through plasma concentration monitoring, if any, and documentation for an optimal plasma concentration range'. This is a rather exceptional situation. If plasma concentration monitoring was applied during the pivotal studies, which should be the case if recommended in the product label, the improved treatment results due to plasma concentration monitoring should be captured in the efficacy criterion.

Risk criteria

Nature and pooling of safety data

Data on adverse effects are generated in clinical trials but for marketed products they result also from post-marketing surveillance reporting. In a number of instances, there might be other sources of data on adverse effects, and in general the following hierarchy of strength of medical evidence is used (1 is the weakest strength and 8 is the most important strength) (Piantadosi, 1995):

1. case reports
2. case series without controls
3. series with literature controls
4. analyses using computer databases
5. case–control studies
6. series based on historical controls
7. single randomized controlled trials
8. combined randomized controlled trials.

In contrast to the efficacy results, the safety data from several controlled clinical trials are usually combined, which provides the highest strength of evidence as noted above. It is therefore recommended that a consistent methodology be used for the data collection and evaluation throughout a clinical trial program (ICH, 1998). Publications exist with regard to the methodology to combine safety data from several clinical trials (Anello and O'Neill, 1996), and the FDA (2003a) has issued a paper which discusses the role of data pooling and appropriate methods for pooling. Used appropriately, pooled analyses can allow detection of relatively rare events, enhance the power to detect a statistical association and protect against chance findings in individual studies, and provide more reliable estimates of the magnitude and constancy of risk over time. Generally, pooled analyses should have the following characteristics: (1) phase I pharmacokinetic and pharmacodynamic studies are excluded; (2) the risk of the safety outcomes of interest are expressed in person-years, or a time-to-event analysis is conducted; (3) the patient population in the pooled analysis is relatively homogeneous with respect to such factors as underlying illness; and (4) a study-specific incidence rate is calculated and compared for any signs of case ascertainment differences.

In the next section, three risk criteria will be established which capture information from the pooled pivotal trials (i.e. overall incidence of adverse effects, overall incidence of serious adverse effects, and discontinuation rate due to adverse effects). In addition, in the following sections the risk criteria 'incidence, seriousness, duration and reversibility of specific adverse effects' and 'safety in subgroups' will be discussed, which capture data from the pooled pivotal trials but also from post-marketing surveillance reporting and possibly other sources. Finally, given that both safety data from clinical trials and safety data from post-marketing surveillance have a number of weaknesses and limitations, which will be discussed in the next sections, a number of criteria are established with regard to the potential for additional risk which has not been forthcoming and demonstrated.

Criteria pertaining to the overall incidence of adverse effects

Arlett stated that it is important to consider the overall adverse reaction profile of a medicine for benefit–risk assessment (Arlett, 2001). Similarly, in Table 2.1 the safety criteria no. 5 ('common and non-serious adverse events'), no. 6 ('serious adverse events'), no. 17 ('deaths') and no. 18 ('incidence of adverse drug reactions') pertain to the incidence of adverse drug effects in general. The FDA (1988) has established three criteria in this respect, which capture the safety data from clinical studies, whether pooled or not, and which are universally applicable to all kind of medicines:

- overall incidence of adverse effects
- overall incidence of serious adverse effects
- discontinuation rate due to adverse effects.

From discussions with several experts in the field it became clear that these criteria are for example very relevant for over the counter (OTC) medicines. OTC medicines have by definition usually only mild side effects, but for such medicines it is very important that the overall incidences of adverse effects and of serious adverse effects are low because they are used widely to treat common ailments.

Also, these three criteria are particularly relevant when the incidences can be put in perspective with the data from the comparator(s) used in the trials (active comparator and/or placebo) (FDA, 2003a). For example, for Zetia (ezetimibe), a cholesterol absorption inhibitor, it is claimed in the US product circular that the incidence of adverse events reported with Zetia was similar to that reported with placebo (Physician's Desk Reference, 2008). Similarly, being able to claim a lower incidence of adverse effects over an active comparator is an important feature of a medicine. Overall incidence of serious adverse effects is probably an even more important parameter to measure safety for most medicines, with 'serious' being defined as resulting in death, being life-threatening, requiring inpatient hospitalization or prolongation of existing hospitalization, resulting in persistent or significant disability/incapacity, or being a congenital anomaly/birth defect (ICH, 1995b). Death can also be considered as a separate criterion as is done by the FDA (see Table 2.1), but it is thought that this is usually not necessary unless there would be a potential mortality issue for a given medicine. Discontinuation rate due to adverse effects (safety criterion no. 22 in Table 2.1) is another criterion that provides an indication with regard to the incidence of significant adverse effects, because it captures situations where either the prescriber or the patient decides that the medicine should be discontinued because of the adverse effect, at the expense of not having the continued benefit of the medicine.

In this section, the term 'adverse effect' (which is the same as 'adverse drug reaction') has been used, which implies a causal relationship to treatment, but it is also possible to use the incidences of 'adverse events', which do not necessarily imply a causal relationship to treatment, for the three above criteria (ICH, 1995b).

Incidence, seriousness, duration and reversibility of specific adverse effects

A number of the safety criteria listed in Table 2.1 pertain to the assessment of specific adverse effects, i.e. the criteria 'similarities and differences in results among studies' (no. 7), 'relation of adverse effects to dose, dose regimen and treatment duration' (no. 9), 'incidence of adverse drug reactions' (no. 18), 'adverse events' (no. 20), and 'laboratory findings, vital signs, electrocardiographs (ECGs)' (no. 21).

Adverse effects or adverse drug reactions are usually divided into two categories (Gruchalla, 2000): reactions that are common, predictable, dose-dependent, related to the pharmacological actions of the medicine, and that may occur in any individual (type A), and reactions that are uncommon, unpredictable, not dose-dependent, usually not related to the pharmacological actions of the medicine, and that occur in susceptible individuals (type B). About 80% of all adverse drug reactions are type A. Type B reactions are often not discovered until after the medicine has been marketed. Both environmental and genetic factors are thought to be important in the development of reactions of this type. Included in this category are drug intolerance, idiosyncratic reactions (i.e. uncharacteristic reactions that are not explicable in terms of the known pharmacological actions of the medicine), and allergic or hypersensitivity reactions.

Whilst in particular the FDA lists clinical adverse effects and laboratory findings/ vital signs/ECGs separately (FDA, 1988), this is usually not done by the European regulatory authorities and in the literature, because clinically relevant deviations from the normal laboratory values are uncommon for most medicines. Laboratory and vital signs adverse effects will therefore not be considered separately in this section, but instead be considered and weighted together with the clinical adverse effects in terms of their incidence, seriousness from a clinical perspective, duration and reversibility.

At the premarketing assessment stage of a new medicine, the safety database consists almost always of data from controlled clinical trials, which are usually pooled as discussed in the previous section. The composition of an appropriate safety database for a new medicine should be determined on a case-by-case basis (FDA, 2003a). Ideally, however, an ideal database should include the following.

- Long-term controlled studies. In most cases, it is preferable to have controlled safety data, to allow for comparisons of event rates and for accurate attribution of adverse events. Control groups could be given a placebo or an active product, depending on the disease being treated. The usefulness of comparators depends on factors such as the background rates of the adverse events of interest. Generally, events that occur rarely and spontaneously (e.g. idiopathic hepatitis) do not need a control group to be interpreted. On the other hand, control groups are essential for detecting changes in rates of events that occur frequently in the population (e.g. death in patients with AD). This is particularly true when the adverse event could be considered part of the disease being treated (e.g. asthma exacerbations occurring with inhalation treatments for asthma).

- A diverse safety database. Ideally, a safety database includes a diverse population which would allow for the development of safety data in important demographic groups such as the elderly, patients with concomitant diseases, or patients taking common concomitant medications.

- Development of safety data over a range of doses. This allows to better characterize the relationship between exposure and the resulting risk, and to provide critical information on the need for dose-adjustments in special populations.

While the product development process is very rigorous, it is not possible to detect all safety concerns during clinical trials. As a result, post-approval safety data collection and risk assessment based on observational data are critical to evaluating and minimizing a product's risk profile (FDA, 2003b). Once a medicine is marketed, there is generally a large increase in the number of patients exposed, including those with comorbid conditions, and those being treated with concomitant medical products. Safety signals identified from case reports (post-marketing surveillance) may be further evaluated in pharmacoepidemiological studies, registries or surveys. Safety signals may be further assessed in terms of their magnitude, the population(s) at risk, changes in risk over time, biologic plausibility, and other factors. Safety signals may provide information about the following:

- new unlabelled adverse events
- an observed increase in the severity or specificity of a labelled event
- an observed increase in the frequency of a labelled event
- new product-product, product-food, or product-dietary supplement interactions
- confusion with a product's name, labelling, packaging or use, either actual or potential.

There are nevertheless a number of challenges with regard to the assessment and interpretation of safety signals:

- calculating the incidence rate and reporting rate; for spontaneous reports, it is not possible to identify all cases due to under-reporting (imprecise numerator), and the size of the exposed population is at best an estimate (imprecise denominator)

- understanding the safety signal with regard to who is at risk and when

- assessing causality.

Overall, assessment of the adverse effects profile of a medicine post-approval involves a complementary review of the safety data from the pre-approval clinical studies, the observational data obtained post-approval (case reports, pharmacoepidemiological studies, registries, surveys), and possibly therapeutic use trials (which may include morbidity/mortality studies and large simple trials which can have as an objective to identify less common adverse effects) (ICH, 1997).

Adverse effects are usually assessed by their incidence, seriousness/severity, and duration (which implies also the outcome as well as the reversibility of the adverse effect) (CIOMS Working Group IV, 1998). However, no standard methods exist for risk weighing of individual adverse effects and for estimating the total risk due to adverse effects (CIOMS Working Group IV, 1998). In this respect, the concept of 'risk driver' (also called the 'dominant risk'), which are the adverse effect(s) that dominate the overall risk profile (carry the most weight), is important to note (CIOMS Working Group IV, 1998). In general, the CIOMS IV report suggests that the three most often reported and the three most serious adverse effects should be chosen as representatives for the risk profile of each medicine, but that all other data on adverse effects should also be taken into account for describing and quantifying the overall risk. Another important concept is that of 'competing risks', and a typical example of this concept was the VIGOR trial with the COX-2 inhibitor rofecoxib (Konstam, 2003), which showed a decrease of serious gastrointestinal adverse effects (perforations, ulcers and bleeds) versus naproxen but at that same time also an increase of myocardial infarctions. This illustrates that weighing competing risks related to different organ systems is challenging. Finally, it is important to note that particular attention should be paid to adverse effects pertaining to hepatotoxicity, because hepatotoxicity has been the most frequent single reason for removing medicines from the market and probably is still the most important single toxicity leading to withdrawal or significant modification of the labelling that may be recognized post-marketing (Temple and Himmel, 2002).

The final aspect which is important in the assessment of specific adverse effects, are methods to prevent, mitigate or manage adverse effects, which can be described in the product label to guide prescribers (safety criterion no. 11 in Table 2.1).

In conclusion, the profile of a medicine with regard to specific adverse effects is undoubtedly the most important criterion within the scope of the assessment of the overall risk profile of a medicine. This is a very comprehensive field, of which the key elements were summarized in this section.

Safety in subgroups

Criterion no. 8 in Table 2.1 pertains to the difference in rate of adverse events in population subgroups. In particular the FDA is very specific in requiring subgroup analyses including demographic subgroup analyses (age, sex, race) and other subgroup analyses (according to body weight, primary diagnosis, secondary diagnosis, concomitant therapy, smoking status and history, and alcohol use) (FDA, 1988, 2003a). According to the FDA, these analyses are critical for the risk assessment, especially the comparison of the adverse effects profile in elderly patients compared to the overall adverse effects profile.

Interactions with other drugs and food

Most medicines have interactions with other medicines and/or food, and therefore the risks for the patient of such interactions should be assessed. The ICH Common Technical Document, the EU Assessment Report and the US Medical Review all three cover interactions as a criterion to be considered (safety criterion no. 15 in Table 2.1). An interaction is usually defined as an alteration either in the pharmacodynamics and/or the pharmacokinetics of a medicine, caused by concomitant drug treatment, dietary factors or social habits such as tobacco or alcohol (CPMP, 1997b). Pharmacodynamic interactions may be caused by a large variety of mechanisms. When similar mechanisms and/or effects are found in animals and in humans, animal studies can be used to characterize a potential interaction. In general, animal, *in vitro* and clinical studies together will describe the pharmacodynamic interaction profile of a medicine. Pharmacokinetic interactions pertain to absorption (P-glycoprotein might be involved in absorption from the gastrointestinal tract), distribution (displacement of drug from plasma proteins), and in particular elimination through metabolic and non-metabolic routes. Metabolism through cytochrome P450 (CYP) enzymes is the reason for many interactions, and a medicine can either be an inducer and/or an inhibitor of one or more CYP450 enzymes (thereby affecting the plasma concentration of other medicines), and/or a substrate (which may cause an effect of the plasma concentration of the medicine if an inhibitor or an inducer of that particular CYP450 enzyme is taken concomitantly). Interactions pertaining to non-metabolic elimination (renal excretion and hepatic/biliary excretion) also occur.

It is important to differentiate between detectable interactions and clinically relevant interactions (CPMP, 1997b). An interaction is clinically relevant when the therapeutic activity and/or toxicity of a medicine is changed to such an extent that a dosage adjustment of the medication or medical intervention may be required, and when concomitant use of two interacting medicines could occur when both are used as therapeutically recommended. Formal interaction studies do however not guarantee a full understanding of all possible risks related to interactions (FDA, 2003a). Ideally, therefore, potential interactions should also be assessed in therapeutic confirmatory trials. One important way unexpected relationships can de detected is by incorporating pharmacokinetic assessments (e.g. population pharmacokinetic studies) in clinical trials, including in safety trials. Finally, safety signals identified from case reports (post-marketing surveillance) might also reveal additional interactions or allow to better characterize known interactions.

Potential for off-label use leading to safety hazards

There can be different kinds of off-label use that can lead to safety hazards:

- use of the medicine outside the indication and/or dosage recommendations (overdose)

- use of the medicine in situations where it is contraindicated (including contraindications during pregnancy and lactation)

- non-compliance with labelled precautions and warnings with regard to interactions, pregnancy and lactation, and driving and operating machines.

A number of the safety criteria listed in Table 2.1 pertain to such off-label use (i.e. criteria no. 12 – 'overdose', no. 16 – 'potential effect on driving and operating machinery', and no. 19 – 'human reproduction data').

As discussed earlier in this chapter, the risk profile of a medicine should be considered within the context of the product label (indication, dosage, contraindications) which establishes the boundaries for the use of the medicine. While it is assumed that physicians will abide by the instructions contained within the label, most physicians regard the label as merely informational, and in fact they are not legally bound by it (Lewis, 1993). This presents somewhat of a problem for regulatory authorities who wish to approve a medicine that may have important safety concerns. A related issue is the off-label use of medicines in children. More than 50% of the medicines used to treat children have not been tested and authorized for use in children (European Commission, 2004). There are several important examples of off-label use which illustrate that it is important to assess and quantify, as a specific risk criterion, the risk for off-label use leading to safety hazards, and to take this into account in determining the overall risk profile of a medicine.

Cerivastatin, an HMG-CoA reductase inhibitor was withdrawn from the market in August 2001 because of cases of rhabdomyolysis. Both the recommendation to start therapy at a lower dose and the warning concerning the interaction with gemfibrozil, which were listed in the product label, were frequently ignored by health professionals, which shows that a risk resulting from frequent off-label use may have significant negative impact on the benefit–risk profile and can eventually lead to withdrawal of the medicine, if the pharmaceutical company fails to stop the off-label use (Schosser, 2002).

Mibefradil, a calcium channel blocker, was withdrawn from the market in June 1998 because of potentially harmful interactions with an unmanageably large number of other medicines. Mibefradil reduced the activity of several CYP450 isoenzymes, most notably 3A4, and therefore interacted with a number of medicines, which was known from both *in vitro* and clinical data prior to approval. Thus, mibefradil's original labelling described hepatic enzyme inhibition and listed the types of medicines with potentially harmful interactions. The FDA strengthened the labelling and issued a public warning after several patients experienced serious adverse events while taking mibefradil with other medications. However, the FDA eventually withdrew mibefradil from the market because it interacted with 26 medicines that were used concomitantly on a common basis, a number and diversity that could not, in practical terms, be addressed by standard labelling instructions or additional public warnings (Friedman *et al.*, 1999).

Isotretinoin, although highly effective for its indication, severe nodular cystic acne, is a known human teratogen causing a range of birth defects. Despite specific labelling and other educational efforts by the manufacturer to prevent exposure during pregnancy, a significant number of foetal exposures still occurred which led the FDA to implement additional measures (Wood, 1999; FDA, 2001).

Potential for non-demonstrated additional risk

It is well known that the safety profile of a medicine is not fully elucidated by the time of its initial approval, and that it might take several years of commercial use and additional therapeutic use clinical studies before all aspects of its safety are fully characterized (Rawlins, 1995). This 'uncertainty' with regard to the safety of a medicine is important to take into account as a specific criterion within the scope of the global risk profile of a medicine, in particular for new medicines. The potential for non-demonstrated additional risks includes non-demonstrated additional safety hazards due to the limitations of clinical trials and/or length of patient exposure, safety issues observed in pre-clinical safety studies but not in humans, and safety issues observed with other drugs of the same pharmacological class. All three aspects are discussed in more detail below.

Potential for non-demonstrated additional risk due to limitations of clinical trials and/or length of patient exposure

It is well recognized that there are a number of limitations with regard to the safety data that are generated in clinical trials – in particular the following.

- The long-term safety beyond the length of exposure in the clinical trials is not established and rare adverse effects are not necessarily detected due to the limited number of patients (Waller, 2001; Hyslop *et al.*, 2002). Safety criteria nos. 4 and 10 in Table 2.1 pertain to this uncertainty. ICH (1995a) has defined the required exposure for medicines intended for long-term treatment of non life-threatening diseases: the total number of patients treated with the medicine should be about 1500, 300 to 600 patients should be treated for 6 months (which should be adequate since most adverse effects first occur and are most frequent within the first few months of treatment), and 100 patients should be treated for a minimum of 1 year (because, although uncommon, some adverse effects may increase in frequency or severity with time, or some serious adverse effects may occur only after treatment of more than six months). However, both ICH and the FDA have established a number of considerations that would suggest the need for a larger database for certain medicines (FDA, 2003a). Irrespectively, it is unlikely that rare serious adverse effects are detected in the pre-approval clinical trials (Kaufman and Shapiro, 2000). In this respect, the 'rule of three' provides guidance that if no events of a particular type are observed, there is a 95% probability that the actual frequency of the event is less than three times the reciprocal of the sample size (Hyslop *et al.*, 2002). Serious adverse effects commonly emerge after approval, so that the safety of new medicines cannot be known with certainty until a medicine has been on the market for many years (Lasser *et al.*, 2002).

- For a number of good reasons, the population included in controlled clinical studies is a restricted group of patients who do not necessarily reflect the standard population who will use the medicine. Patients with comorbidity and patients taking concomitant medications might be excluded from the trials, which has as a consequence that there might be uncertainty with regard to the safety and drug interactions in a 'real world' setting (Hyslop *et al.*, 2002; Simon, 2002).

Even when a product is on the market, its full safety profile might not be known because, as noted above, it takes several years to establish all safety aspects of a medicine. This is also one of the reasons why the ICH Common Technical Document considers worldwide marketing experience as an important safety criterion (safety criterion no. 13 in Table 2.1). In addition, case reports, which are the cornerstone of pharmacovigilance for the detection of unanticipated adverse effects, have a number of limitations (Kaufman and Shapiro, 2000). Case reports are generally written about rare or striking events, or events that immediately follow the start of therapy (e.g. anaphylaxis). Case reports alone have raised many suspicions, and are occasionally sufficient to establish very strong associations, especially if there are numerous reports linking rare exposures to rare outcomes (e.g. anabolic steroids and liver tumours), or repeat episodes of an event after re-challenge. However, in most instances, case reports are insufficient by themselves to document associations, and still less to establish causality, because there is no comparison group to allow for a quantitative estimate of risk, and frequently not even a reliable denominator of users from which an incidence rate can be estimated. In addition, once a suspicion has been widely publicized, physicians could tend to report cases exposed to that medicine but not cases that occur among users of other medicines or no medicine at all. This can lead to biased conclusions. In addition, there is usually no assessment of the possibility that an apparent association may be explained by factors other than the medicine at issue. Finally, associations between medicines and common or delayed outcomes are seldom the subject of case reports, because they are difficult to discern at the individual level. Despite these limitations, case reports have often served as the only source of information about serious adverse effects.

Safety issues observed in preclinical safety studies but not in humans

It is conceivable that, for a given medicine, safety issues are observed in preclinical studies and not (yet) in humans, but which might in theory be relevant for patients. Therefore, it is warranted to take such pre-clinical safety issues into account as a potential risk, consistent with the ICH Common Technical Document (safety criterion no. 3 in Table 2.1). An example of a preclinical safety finding is cataract which was observed in female rats and in dogs with simvastatin but not in humans, and which is mentioned in the product label for Zocor under Precautions because of its potential relevance for patients (Physician's Desk Reference, 2008).

Safety issues observed with other medicines of the same pharmacological class

A specific safety criterion on this subject originating from the ICH Common Technical Document is listed in Table 2.1 (criterion no. 1). It is possible that some of the safety features of other medicines in the same pharmacological class could also be relevant for the medicine in question, in particular if the other medicine(s) in the class has generated a more comprehensive clinical program and/or more data from post-marketing surveillance. Despite the fact that there is little validity and/or precedent for a so-called 'class effect' with regard to the safety of medicines with similar or even identical mechanisms of action (Dujovne, 2002), for determining the risk profile of a medicine it is appropriate taking into account, as a precautionary measure, significant safety issues seen with other products of the same class but not identified with the medicine in question. Such safety issues should be considered as 'uncertainty factors' until their relevance for the subject medicine is fully established.

Dismissed risk (safety) criteria

The following two safety criteria listed in Table 2.1 were dismissed because they do not have a specific impact on the risk of a medicine within the scope of the prerequisites defined earlier in this chapter.

- Safety criterion no. 2 – 'special approaches to monitoring for particular adverse events'. Whilst monitoring for specific adverse events might enhance the likelihood of characterizing those adverse events, it has no direct impact on the safety profile of a medicine. The FDA Clinical Review lists in addition a number of specific areas to which attention should be paid, i.e. immunogenicity for monoclonal antibodies, the effect on growth for medicines for children, human carcinogenicity for medicines for chronic use, and QTc prolongation. If there would be a valid concern in any of those areas, it can be taken into account within the scope of the previously defined general safety criteria 'incidence, seriousness, duration and reversibility of specific adverse effects' and 'potential for non-demonstrated additional risk'.

- Safety criterion no. 14 – 'support for the applicability to a specific region of data generated in another region'. This is an ICH criterion which is of particular significance in Japan, since most medicines are first developed and filed for registration in Europe and the United States.

2.4 VERIFICATION OF THE LIST OF BENEFIT AND RISK CRITERIA BY MEANS OF A SURVEY

The list of benefit and risk criteria which was identified and discussed in the previous section was further checked by means of a questionnaire for experts in the field, who were asked to indicate for each benefit and risk criterion if in their view it should be taken into account in a model for benefit–risk assessment. The purpose of this questionnaire was to have an initial very general confirmation of the validity of each criterion.

A questionnaire was sent to all participants of the workshop organized by CMR International Institute for Regulatory Science on 'Risk Management: The role of Regulatory Strategies in the Development of New Medicines', which took place on April 25–26 2002 (Workshop review, 2002). The questionnaire was sent out by CMR International Institute before the workshop and results were collected prior to the workshop. The workshop was attended by invitation by senior people from the regulatory authorities (11 attendees) and from the pharmaceutical industry (28 attendees). People were asked to indicate which of the safety and efficacy criteria listed in the questionnaire should, in their opinion, be included in a model for benefit–risk assessment.

Table 2.2 lists the results of the questionnaire. The vast majority of responders (between 70 and 100%) indicated that each of the listed efficacy criteria, with the exception of 'anticipated patient compliance', should be included in a model. The views with regard to 'anticipated patient compliance' were more divergent since overall 55% of responders indicated that this criterion should be included in a model, although all (seven) responders from the regulatory authorities confirmed the need for this criterion. The results for the risk criteria were very similar, and with the exception of 'potential safety risks with off-label use', the vast majority (between 75 and 100%) of the responders were of the opinion that each of the listed risk criteria should be included in a model. Nevertheless, a smaller majority (60%) of responders, equally split between responders from authorities and responders from industry, considered that 'potential safety risks with off-label use' should be included in a model.

There were however some differences between the list of criteria and the terms used for each criterion in the previous sections of this chapter, and the list included in the questionnaire, which originated from the fact that the list of criteria was further refined and completed following the completion of the survey in April 2002. The most significant differences were that in the questionnaire 'efficacy versus comparator' was split into two criteria ('magnitude of the treatment effect' and 'clinical relevance of the magnitude of the treatment effect'), 'efficacy as per the results of the non-primary endpoints' and 'efficacy as per the results of relevant non-pivotal trials and extensions' were taken together in one criterion, 'clustering (consistency) of results

Table 2.2   Results of the questionnaire on the inclusion of benefit and risk criteria in a model for benefit–risk assessment

	Total number[a] (% of responders) who considered that the criterion should be included in a model[b]
Benefit criteria	
Magnitude of the treatment effect (obtained from the results of the primary endpoints in the pivotal clinical trials)	20 (7 + 13) (100)
Clinical relevance of the magnitude of the treatment effect	20 (7 + 13) (100)
Statistical significance of the treatment effect	18 (7 + 11) (90)
Relevance of the primary endpoints of the pivotal clinical trials	19 (7 + 12) (95)
Relevance of the studied population of the pivotal clinical trials	18 (7 + 11) (90)
Evidence for the efficacy in relevant subgroups in the pivotal clinical trials	14 (7 + 7) (70)
Statistical/design robustness of the pivotal clinical trials	18 (7 + 11) (90)
Confirmation of treatment effect by results of secondary endpoints and results of non-pivotal trials	16 (6 + 10) (80)
Anticipated patient compliance	11 (7 + 4) (55)
Risk criteria	
Overall incidence of adverse effects (from clinical trials)	16 (5 +11) (80)
Overall incidence of serious adverse effects (from clinical trials)	20 (7 + 13) (100)
Discontinuation rate due to adverse effects (from clinical trials)	15 (5 + 10) (75)
Incidence, seriousness and duration of specific adverse effects (from clinical trials and post-marketing surveillance)	20 (7 + 13) (100)
Interactions with other drugs and with food	18 (7 + 11) 90 %
Safety in subgroups (e.g. age, race, sex)	20 (7 +13) (100)
Potential safety risks with off-label use	12 (4 + 8) (60)
Generaliability of the safety profile to the general population	18 (7 + 11) (90)

[a]Split by regulatory authorities and industry.
[b]$N = 20$; 7 from regulatory authorities and 13 from industry.

of the pivotal trials' was missing, and the three criteria pertaining to the potential for non-demonstrated additional risk were reflected in one criterion entitled 'general-iability of the safety profile to the general population'.

Despite these differences and the fact this was a very simple questionnaire which should be considered as exploratory, the overall results confirmed that in general the list of benefit and risk criteria was adequate and that none of the listed criteria should be dismissed. In a subsequent CMR workshop in 2008, the above benefit and risk criteria were further reviewed, refined and elaborated. The conclusions of this workshop including the revised list of criteria can be found in Chapter 6.

CHAPTER 3

Review of the Current Benefit–Risk Assessment Models

3.1 BACKGROUND

The purpose of this chapter is to describe and review in detail the existing models for benefit–risk assessment of medicines. An extensive literature search was conducted with the purpose to find all publications which describe a model for benefit–risk assessment, in particular a model that is able to take into account all available evidence for the benefit and risk of a given medicine. In addition, experts in the field of benefit–risk assessment were consulted and asked about the models of which they were aware. Finally, the available models were also discussed during several external presentations (Mussen, 2001, 2002) and with many colleagues in the pharmaceutical industry.

The main focus of this chapter is on models which aim at taking into account the full available safety and efficacy data from multiple clinical trials and from post-marketing safety data of a given medicine. In addition to these models, there are also many methods and models that aim at establishing the safety and efficacy data of a single clinical trial into a benefit–risk balance or ratio. Other models that exist are those that have been developed for specific products, or specific classes of products, and that are able to integrate the specific outcomes attributed to these products. A brief overview of the most important of the latter two kinds of models will be provided in this chapter, since some of them contain useful ideas for the development of a new model for benefit–risk assessment.

Three general models for benefit–risk assessment of medicines are reviewed in this chapter: (1) the 'Principle of Threes' grading system (Edwards *et al.*, 1996); (2) the TURBO model (CIOMS Working Group IV, 1998); and (3) the Evidence-based Benefit and Risk Model (Beckmann, 1999). The first two methods are also described in the

Benefit-Risk Appraisal of Medicines Filip Mussen, Sam Salek, Stuart Walker
© 2009 John Wiley & Sons, Ltd

Report of the CIOMS Working Group IV entitled 'Benefit–risk Balance for Marketed Drugs: Evaluating Safety Signals' (CIOMS Working Group IV, 1998). All three models have been developed either within the scope of the evaluation of the benefit–risk balance of marketed products because of a safety concern, and/or by people who are primarily involved in pharmacovigilance activities. The primary focus of these models is therefore more on safety than efficacy, and more on the re-evaluation of marketed medicines than the evaluation of new medicines. The models are reviewed below in terms of background, concept, purpose, description, and application, followed by a discussion of their strengths and weaknesses. They are also analysed with regard to the incorporation of the 10 benefit criteria and the 10 risk criteria that were identified in Chapter 2 as being relevant for models for benefit–risk assessment:

- Benefit Criteria

  ► Efficacy versus comparator and its clinical relevance (for each pivotal trial)

  ► Design, conduct and statistical adequacy of the trial (for each pivotal trial)

  ► Clinical relevance of the primary endpoints (for each pivotal trial)

  ► Representativeness of the studied population for the population targeted in the label (for each pivotal trial)

  ► Statistical significance of the efficacy results (for each pivotal trial)

  ► Evidence for the efficacy in relevant subgroups (for each pivotal trial)

  ► Efficacy as per the results of the non-primary endpoints (for each pivotal trial)

  ► Efficacy as per the results of the relevant non-pivotal trials and extensions

  ► Anticipated patient compliance in market use

  ► Clustering (consistency) of results of the pivotal trials

- Risk Criteria

  ► Overall incidence of adverse effects

  ► Overall incidence of serious adverse effects

  ► Discontinuation rate due to adverse effects

  ► Incidence, seriousness, duration and reversibility of specific adverse effects

  ► Safety in subgroups

▶ Interactions with other drugs and food

▶ Potential for off-label use leading to safety hazards

▶ Potential for non-demonstrated additional risk due to limitations of clinical trials and/or length of patient exposure

▶ Potential for non-demonstrated additional risk due to safety issues observed in preclinical safety studies but not in humans

▶ Potential for non-demonstrated additional risk due to safety issues observed with other medicines of the same pharmacological class.

The question that is addressed is how closely these models match the ideal model that would take into account all these benefit and risk criteria. As such, this evaluation serves as a face validity testing which is concerned with the extent to which the contents of a method look like they are measuring what they are supposed to measure (The School of Community, Health Sciences and Social Care, 2000).

3.2 EVALUATION OF THE EXISTING BENEFIT–RISK ASSESSMENT MODELS

The 'Principle of Threes' grading system

Background, concept and purpose of the model

Edwards *et al.* (1996) set out to establish a simple and quick methodology to evaluate the benefit–risk balance of a medicine. The model is based upon the concepts of 'seriousness', 'duration' and 'incidence' as related to disease indication, disease amelioration by a medicine, and the adverse effects ascribed to the medicine. The questions which Edwards *et al.* tried to address by developing this model were: (1) whether the use of a simple algorithm or quantified method for risk and benefit calculation could provide some insights into how we think about the risks and benefits of medicines; and (2) whether it is possible to develop a tool that will enable a first rough assessment of a medicine to be made and possibly even help make comparisons between medicines?

Description of the model

An overview of the 'Principle of Threes' grading system is provided in Table 3.1. As mentioned above, the model establishes the concepts of seriousness, duration

Table 3.1   'Principle of Threes' grading system

	High	Medium	Low
Disease			
Seriousness			
Duration			
Incidence			
Level of improvement produced by the medicine			
Seriousness			
Duration			
Incidence			
Adverse effects of the medicine			
Seriousness			
Duration			
Incidence			

and incidence as related to disease indication, disease amelioration by a medicine, and the adverse effects ascribed to the medicine. Each parameter is rated as high, medium or low. The methodology is essentially based on the visible weighing of the scores for the 'level of improvement produced by the medicine' against the scores for the 'adverse effects' criteria. A third dimension, i.e. the seriousness, duration and incidence of disease, is used to determine how much the benefit must outweigh the risks.

Definitions for grading the disease parameters are also proposed (Table 3.2).

Table 3.2   Grading system for disease

	High	Medium	Low
Seriousness	Fatal	Disabling	Inconvenient
Duration	Permanent	Persistent	Temporary
Incidence	Common	Frequent	Rare

It is assumed that, normally, all patients who take a medicine have the disease for which the medicine is indicated. Therefore, as for the disease parameter, the incidence is usually graded as high. However, for medicines used for prophylaxis the disease incidence is graded as low. Similarly, the incidence of the level of improvement produced by the medicine is low for prophylactic medicines.

As for the adverse effects to be taken into consideration in the grading system, Edwards *et al.* proposed to consider the three most common and the three most serious adverse effects. It is argued that this choice is arbitrary but practical; the frequency of the three most common adverse effects gives an indication of the frequency of the other adverse effects, and similarly the seriousness of the three most serious adverse effects provides a limit for the seriousness of the other adverse effects.

Nevertheless, Edward *et al.* mentioned that it is important that the total profile of adverse drug effects is considered and that the arguments for the selection of the representative reactions are clearly stated. Deviations from considering the three most common and the three most serious adverse effects should be fully justified. Possible arguments are that: (1) a medicine might have several other common adverse effects; (2) the exact frequencies of the adverse effects are not known, so that discrimination cannot be made on the basis of incidence; and (3) a medicine that is associated with a large number of adverse effects should have a worse estimate of risk than one associated with only a few.

Application of the model

In the Report of the CIOMS Working Group IV, the model was applied to three examples (felbamate, dipyrone, and quinine) to illustrate its applicability. A numerical scale was used for the qualitative terms as follows: low = 1; medium = 2; high = 3; no effect/no influence = 0. This scale facilitates the assessment of the trade-off between benefit and risks.

Example: felbamate

Felbamate is the only effective treatment for Lennox–Gastaut epilepsy, a disease with high mortality (1 in 500), and thus seriousness of disease was rated as 'high'. The disease is intractable (duration permanent, which equals 'high') and rare (400 cases per year in France; incidence = rare). Felbamate reduces dramatically the morbidity and mortality of Lennox–Gastaut epilepsy (seriousness and duration of the level of improvement produced by the medicine are both 'high'), but has no influence on the natural course of the disease since it suppresses rather than prevents or cures it (incidence score = 0).

Blood dyscrasia with aplastic anaemia is the adverse effect driving the risk profile. The seriousness of the adverse effect is 'high', the duration generally persistent ('medium'), and the incidence is estimated at 1 in 4000 treated patients ('medium' incidence).

In summary, this provides the following grading:

	Disease	Effectiveness of the medicine	Dominant reaction
Seriousness	3	3	3
Duration	3	3	2
Incidence	1	0	2
TOTAL	7	6	7

Thus, according to this rating, the dominant adverse reaction risk profile is similar to the disease profile and marginally worse than the effectiveness of the medicine. However, the regulatory authorities decided in this particular case, for a disease for which no other effective treatment exists, that such an effective medicine as felbamate could be used for this special population but was not suitable for the general treatment of epilepsy.

Example: dipyrone

Dipyrone is a non-narcotic analgesic that has no anti-inflammatory action. It is used for the treatment of fever and pain. Agranulocytosis is considered as the dominant risk for this medicine. Scores were attributed as follows:

	Disease	Effectiveness of the medicine	Dominant reaction
Seriousness	1	3	3
Duration	1	3	2
Incidence	3	0	1
TOTAL	5	6	6

These scores do not allow making an obvious judgement between the effects of the disease, the effectiveness of the medicine and the dominant adverse effect. As a comparison, the 'principle of threes' grading system was also applied to aspirin, for which the dominant risk was considered to be gastrointestinal bleeding. The scores are as follows:

	Disease	Effectiveness of the medicine	Dominant reaction
Seriousness	1	3	3
Duration	1	3	2
Incidence	3	0	2
TOTAL	5	6	7

Surprisingly, the relatively high incidence of gastrointestinal bleeding associated with aspirin gives a better risk profile to dipyrone than to aspirin, although the safety of dipyrone has been the subject of extensive discussions and proposed measures, including its withdrawal from the market.

Example: quinine

Quinine was indicated for the treatment of nocturnal leg cramps and had over-the-counter status in the United States. Limited data from clinical trials in this indication were available and these data did not support the efficacy of quinine in this indication. Thrombocytopenia (thr) and arrhythmia (arr) were considered to be the risk drivers. The scores are as follows according to the CIOMS IV report:

	Disease	Effectiveness of the medicine	Dominant reaction
Seriousness	1	1 (or 0)	2 (thr), 1(arr)
Duration	1	1 (or 0)	2 (thr), 1 (arr)
Incidence	2	0	1 (thr), 1 (arr)
TOTAL	4	2 (or 0)	4.0 (mean)

These results show that quinine was ineffective (score of 2) for this relatively trivial condition (score of 4). Although the score for the adverse effects was relatively low (3 for thrombocytopenia and 5 for arrhythmia), the benefit–risk balance is unfavourable.

In 1995, this indication was withdrawn because quinine was considered to be no longer safe and effective for the treatment of leg cramps, although it remains available in the United Kingdom for this indication.

Quantitative approach

The above semiquantitative model for assessing benefit–risk was modified to a quantitative model in the Report of the CIOMS Working Group IV. The rationale provided in the CIOMS IV Report for changing the model to a quantitative model is that it could be useful when sufficient data on both benefits and risks are available. The proposed scoring system is as follows:

Benefit score = cure rate × seriousness of the disease × chronicity/duration of the disease

Cure rate = rate (fraction) of responders

Seriousness of the disease:	High (fatal): score = 30
	Medium (disabling): score = 20
	Low (inconvenient): score = 10
Chronicity/duration of the disease:	High (permanent) = 30
	Medium (persistent) = 20
	Low (temporary) = 10

Score for each adverse effect = incidence × seriousness × duration

Incidence=trate fraction of patients that had the adverse effect

Seriousness:	High: score = 30
	Medium: score = 20
	Low: score = 10
Duration:	High: score = 30
	Medium: score = 20
	Low: score = 10

Scores are calculated for the three most common adverse effects and for the three most serious adverse effects. The risk score is the average score of these six values. The overall benefit–risk ratio is then calculated by dividing the benefit score by the risk score. Compared to the original semiquantitative model, the criteria 'seriousness of the level of improvement produced by the medicine', 'duration of the level of improvement produced by the medicine', and 'incidence of the disease' were omitted, but no reasons were given for these omissions. It is in particular incomprehensible why the first two criteria were ignored and how the effectiveness of a medicine can be characterized solely by the rate (fraction) of responders (which is called the 'cure rate'). Furthermore, the term 'cure rate' is inaccurate since not all medicines 'cure' a disease.

No real-life examples of this quantitative model have been described in the literature. Therefore, in an effort to try to illustrate the applicability of this model, the model was used to calculate the benefit–risk balance of two different kinds of medicines:

- the ACE inhibitor enalapril, for the treatment of congestive heart failure, a potentially life-threatening disease

- the 5-HT$_{1B/1D}$ agonist rizatriptan for the treatment of migraine, a non-life threatening disease.

Example of the quantitative approach: enalapril

The SOLVD trial (The SOLVD Investigators, 1991), a mega-trial involving 2569 patients, demonstrated that enalapril significantly reduces mortality and hospitalization for heart failure in patients with chronic congestive heart failure and low ejection fractions. At the end of the scheduled follow-up of the study (on average 41.4 months), 39.7% of patients had died in the placebo group compared with 35.2% of patients in the enalapril group (relative risk reduction of 16%, 95% confidence interval 5–26%, $p = 0.0036$). 57.3% of patients died or were hospitalized for worsening of congestive heart failure, as compared with 47.7% of patients in the enalapril group (relative risk reduction of 26%, 95% confidence interval 18–34%, $p < 0.0001$). In the enalapril group, there was significantly more dizziness or fainting (57%), which are indicative of hypotension, versus the placebo group (50%), and cough (37% versus 31%), but there was no excess of angioedema (3.8% in the enalapril group versus 4.1% in the placebo group).

The 'cure rate' can be considered as being 0.648 (100 – 35.2% of the patients who had died at the end of the follow-up period), although it should be recognized that this assumption ignores the 'cure rate' of 0.603 in the placebo group (100 – 39.7%). The seriousness of congestive heart failure is fatal and this can thus be assumed to correspond to the highest score which is 30. The chronicity/duration of the disease is permanent and again presumably corresponds to the highest score of 30. The benefit score is thus 583.2 ($0.648 \times 30 \times 30$).

From the above description of the study results it can be concluded that dizziness or fainting and cough are the main risk drivers, and therefore scores for both adverse effects were calculated. Assuming that in the SOLVD trial the excess incidence of dizziness or fainting was 7% (0.07), its seriousness medium (score $= 20$), and its duration low (score $= 10$) (Physician's Desk Reference, 2008), the risk score for hypotension is 14. The excess incidence of cough was 0.06, its seriousness low (score $= 10$), and its duration high (score $= 30$) (Physician's Desk Reference, 2008). The risk score for cough is thus 18, and the average risk score of both adverse effects 16.

The overall benefit–risk ratio is thus $583.2/16 = 36.5$.

Example of the quantitative approach: rizatriptan

The efficacy of rizatriptan in the acute treatment of migraine attacks was established in four placebo-controlled trials (Physician's Desk Reference, 2008). Headache relief occurred starting 30 min following dosing, and response rates (i.e. reduction of moderate or severe headache pain to no or mild pain) 2 h after treatment were 67–77% with the recommended dose of 10 mg compared to 23–40% with placebo. The most common side effects are dizziness, somnolence and asthenia/fatigue (incidences between 5 and 10%). The most serious but very rare side effects associated with the use of rizatriptan and other triptans are myocardial ischemia or infarction, and cerebrovascular accident.

Assuming that on average 72% (0.72) of patients experienced pain relief (i.e. the average between 67 and 77%) and can thus considered as being responders, that the seriousness of migraine is disabling (score = 20), and that the duration is temporary (score = 10), the benefit score equals 144 (i.e. $0.72 \times 10 \times 20$).

The three most common side effects are dizziness, somnolence and asthenia/fatigue. Their incidence is conservatively assumed to be 10% (0.1), and their seriousness and duration both low (score = 10), which corresponds to a risk score of 10 (i.e. $0.1 \times 10 \times 10$). All three side effects have thus the same risk score. The three most serious side effects are myocardial ischaemia and infarction, and cerebrovascular accident. These three side effects occur very rarely and for the sake of this exercise it is assumed that 'very rarely' corresponds to an incidence of 0.001% (European Commission, 1999), but they have obviously the highest scores for seriousness and duration. This corresponds to a risk score of 0.009 for each of these three side effects (i.e. $0.00001 \times 30 \times 30$). The average overall risk score which averages the score of all six side effects is thus 5.0045. The risk score is thus almost exclusively determined by the three rather frequent but innocent side effects, and not by three rare but potentially very serious side effects.

The overall benefit–risk ratio is thus $144/5.0045 = 28.8$.

Strengths and weaknesses of the model

Strengths of the model

The main strength of the 'Principle of Threes' model is that it takes into account the seriousness of the disease, because this allows the opportunity to quantify how much the benefit must outweigh the risks. This can be illustrated with two extreme examples: an OTC medicine to treat heartburn and an anticancer medicine. Assuming that both medicines are equally effective in the disease for which they are indicated (seriousness, duration and incidence of the level of improvement produced by the medicine rated as 'high'), the safety profile of the OTC medicine must be much more favourable than the safety profile of the anticancer medicine, which generally includes a number of serious adverse effects, because no prescriber or patient would accept a significant risk for serious adverse effects for an OTC medicine to treat heartburn. Thus, on a theoretical basis, the intrinsic benefit of the OTC medicine must outweigh its risks to a much greater extent than should be the case for the anticancer medicine. Taking into account the seriousness of the disease compensates into the equation of benefit versus risk the fact that for medicines for serious diseases it is generally allowed that the benefits outweigh the risks to a lesser extent than for non-serious diseases.

The other advantage of this model is that it is very simple and allows making a quick but very crude assessment of the benefit–risk profile of a medicine.

Weaknesses of the model

The model described by Edwards *et al.* (1996) includes several important weaknesses:.

- The model covers essentially only one of the benefit criteria established in Chapter 2 (i.e. 'efficacy versus comparator and its clinical relevance') and one of the risk criteria (i.e. 'incidence, seriousness and duration of specific adverse effects') but ignores all other criteria.

- The grading system is not well-defined, i.e. when a score of 'high', 'medium' or 'low' should be assigned, and having three scores only does not necessarily allow sufficient discrimination. For example, if the incidence of the level of improvement produced by the medicine or the incidence of the adverse effects of the medicine is expressed as high, medium or low, this will only provide a very crude idea of the magnitude of the actual incidence. Second, it is not obvious what high, medium, and low represent for each of the nine parameters. The model could be significantly improved if the grading systems for the level of improvement and for the adverse effect could be defined, similar to the work done for the grading system for the disease (see Table 3.2). However, the statement by Edwards that the level of improvement produced by prophylactic medicines should be graded as low is certainly controversial. It can be argued that vaccines that provide an immunization against potentially serious infectious diseases in usually close to 100% of patients should be graded as 'high' in terms of seriousness and incidence of the level of improvement produced by the vaccine.

- It is highly questionable whether the incidence of the disease should be taken into account for any benefit–risk assessment of a given medicine. For example, the benefit–risk assessment of a highly effective and safe medicine for an orphan indication should not be influenced by the fact that the disease is very rare. In this respect, it should be noted that the quantitative approach derived from the descriptive model developed by Edwards does not take incidence of disease into account.

- With regard to the adverse effects, Edwards *et al.* argued that the three most common and the three most serious adverse effects should be considered. However, their paper lacks a sound rationale for this proposal. The CIOMS IV Report mentions as well that as a first step the three most often reported and the three most serious adverse reactions should be chosen as representative for the risk profile of a medicine, but again no further justification is provided for this approach. It is unclear whether there has been any research pertaining to the thesis that the three most common and the three most serious adverse effects are an accurate representation of the overall safety profile of a medicine. A literature search did not reveal any pertinent publications on this subject. Edwards *et al.* recognized that flexibility might be required and they state that the selection of the adverse effects should be argued in each individual case. In this respect it should be noted that in the examples listed in the CIOMS IV Report and discussed above (felbamate, dipyrone, quinine) one or two risk drivers were listed.

- Judgement with regard to the type, quality and relative importance of the data (e.g. safety data from clinical trials versus safety data from spontaneous reporting) is required because data can be different in terms of these three criteria, but this judgement cannot be taken into account to fill in the cells in the model. This is an inherent issue of this model as pointed out by Edwards *et al.* themselves.

- The model has not been validated and its actual use seems to be very limited.

The quantitative approach described in the CIOMS IV report includes three major flaws which, taken together, exclude that this model can be used to calculate a benefit–risk ratio that would accurately represent the actual benefit–risk profile of a given medicine. First, in the algorithm for the benefit score, the efficacy of the medicine is only taken into account through the 'cure rate', which is defined as the fraction of responders. The magnitude of the clinical effect is thus not considered. For example, a medicine with a very modest clinical effect in 100% of patients would thus have a benefit score which would be twice as high as the benefit score of a medicine with a clinically very significant effect in 50% of patients but no significant effect in the other patients. Not taking into account the clinical significance of the magnitude of the effect of a medicine is inappropriate, as discussed in Chapter 2.

The second major flaw is that the possible scores 'high' (30), 'medium' (20), and 'low' (10) for seriousness of the disease, chronicity/duration of the disease, seriousness of an adverse effect, and duration of an adverse effect seem to be arbitrary and any justification and validation for these scores has not been provided. Lastly, the risk score is almost exclusively driven by the frequent adverse effects. In contrast, any rare but serious adverse effects do not significantly contribute to the overall risk score. As illustrated in the above example on rizatriptan, the incidence of an adverse effect is the driver of the risk score, since it can vary in practice between 0.01% (or less) and

10% (a factor of 1000), whilst the scores for seriousness and duration can only vary between 10 and 30. Most rare adverse effects, and even life-threatening ones, will always have a very low risk score due to their low incidence, as compared to the more frequent (but usually less serious) adverse effects.

Overall, both the descriptive model and the quantitative model have certain merits but important weaknesses prevent their proper use at present. Further development and ultimately validation of this model are required.

The TURBO model

Background, concept and purpose of the model

The TURBO ('Transparent Uniform Risk/Benefit Overview') model is a quantitative and graphical approach to benefit–risk analysis, developed by Amery and described in the CIOMS Working Group IV Report (1998). This method tries to quantify the benefits and risks (i.e. the benefit factor B and the risk factor R) of a medicine in a given indication, and both factors are then displayed on the TURBO diagram. Very little information is provided in the CIOMS IV Report with regard to the rationale and underlying principles of this model. Its main objective is to place each medicine in an XY benefit–risk diagram. According to the author, the TURBO-diagram provides a composite for between-drug comparisons.

Description of the model

The risk factor 'R' is defined as the sum of R_0 and R_C, where R_0 is the risk associated with the medically most serious adverse effect, and where R_C represents the additional risk, that is, the next most serious adverse effect or, if there is no next most serious adverse effect, the most frequent adverse effect. The R_0 score is calculated by quantifying the frequency and severity of the most serious adverse effect in a diagram and then selecting the corresponding score (Table 3.3). The score for R_0 can range from 1 to 5, and the score for R_C from 0 to 2 (see below).

Table 3.3 Calculating the R-score associated with the most serious adverse effect (R_0)

Estimated attributable risk		Minor	Slight	Moderate	Severe	Very severe
	Frequent	2 (?)				5
	Common				4	
	Not uncommon			3		
	Rare		2			
	Very rare	1				3 (?)
				Estimated severity		

This model was not yet fully developed at the time of publication and therefore scores were not attributed to all cells, or question marks were put with some of the scores.

Tentative definitions were proposed for the five categories pertaining to severity:

Minor = some hindrance, but not really incapacitating

Slight = temporarily/intermittently incapacitating

Moderate = incapacitating, but not life-threatening or life-shortening

Severe = life-shortening, but not life-threatening

Very severe = life-threatening.

The R_C score is calculated as follows.

- Estimate the R-score (Table 3.3) for the next most serious adverse effect or, if there is no next most serious adverse effect, the most frequent adverse effect; this is the R' score.

- If $R' = 5$, then $R_C = 2$
  If $R' = 4$, then $R_C = 1$
  If $R' \leq 3$, then $R_C = 0$.

The R-factor is thus the sum of R_0 and R_C, and can thus vary between 1 ($R_0 = 1$ and $R_C = 0$) and 7 ($R_0 = 5$ and $R_C = 2$).

The Benefit factor B is calculated in a similar way as the R-factor and is defined as the sum of B_0 and B_C, where B_0 is the primary benefit and B_C the ancillary benefit. The B_0 score, which ranges from 1 to 5, is calculated by quantifying the probability of benefit and the degree of benefit in a diagram and then selecting the corresponding score (Table 3.4).

This model was not yet fully developed at the time of publication and therefore scores were not attributed to all cells.

Table 3.4 Calculating the B-score associated with the benefit in the given indication (B_0)

Probability		Minor	Slight	Moderate	Marked	Major
of benefit	Nearly always					5
	Frequent				4	
	Common			3		
	Not uncommon		2			
	Rare	1				
		Minor	Slight	Moderate	Marked	Major
				Degree of benefit		

Tentative definitions were proposed for the five categories pertaining to estimating the degree of benefit:

Minor = the treated condition becomes less hindering, but capabilities remain unchanged

Slight = the treated condition becomes less frequently incapacitating or incapability lasts shorter

Moderate = the treated condition becomes less incapacitating, but no change in life expectancy

Marked = the treated condition becomes less life-shortening

Major = the treated condition becomes less immediately life-threatening.

The B_C score is estimated as follows.

- $B_C = 2$ if ancillary *medical* property exists relevant to the indication (e.g. cholesterol-lowering effect for antidiabetic medicine).

- $B_C = 1$ if ancillary *practical* property exists (e.g. once-daily dosage schedule or fast onset of action).

The R-factor and the B-factor are placed in the TURBO diagram (which includes benefit on the X-axis and risk on the Y-axis), and a T-score which is also called the intrinsic risk–benefit balance and which ranges from 1 to 7, is assigned (Table 3.5). According to Amery, the T-scores had to be further defined, and in the CIOMS IV publication T-scores were not attributed to all cells.

Table 3.5 The TURBO diagram

R-factor							
7	T = 1	T = 2	T = 3				T = 4
6						T = 4	
5					T = 4		T = 7
4				T = 4		T = 6	
3			T = 4			T = 5	
2		T = 4					
1	T = 4						
	1	2	3	4	5	6	7	B-factor

Application of the model

There are no real-life examples in the literature which describe the benefit–risk profile of a medicine according to this model. Therefore, in an effort to try to illustrate the actual use of the model, it was applied to the same two medicines which were used as an example for the quantitative 'Principle of Threes' model:

- the ACE inhibitor enalapril, for the treatment of congestive heart failure, a potentially life-threatening disease

- the 5-HT$_{1B/1D}$ agonist rizatriptan for the treatment of migraine, a non-life threatening disease.

Example: enalapril

The properties of enalapril in terms of its key safety and efficacy data have been described in the section on the 'Principle of Threes' model. The probability of benefit, that is, the percentage of patients in which life is prolonged, can be estimated as 'common'. Although no definitions are provided by the author with regard to the five categories for the probability for benefit (nearly always, frequent, common, not uncommon, rare) a 16% reduction in risk can be considered arbitrarily as common. The degree of benefit corresponds to 'marked', since heart failure becomes less life-shortening. Although no score has been attributed to the corresponding cell in the table for calculating the B-score, a B-score of 3.5 seems logical. It is considered that enalapril has no ancillary medical or practical properties that would warrant a B$_C$ score. The potentially medically most serious adverse effect associated with the use of enalapril in the SOLVD trial was dizziness or fainting, which are indicative of hypotension. Since the incidence of dizziness or fainting was 57% in the enalapril group versus 50% in the placebo group, the attributable risk can be considered as 'common' if it is assumed that the definition of 'common' corresponds with the definition for this term established in the CIOMS III report (1% and <10%) (CIOMS Working Group III, 1995). The estimated severity can be considered as 'slight', which is defined as temporarily/ intermittently incapacitating, and which is realistic if the initiation of treatment and dose increases are well managed (Physician's Desk Reference, 2008). As shown in Table 3.3, a score of 3 can be assigned for R$_0$, but this score is an estimate since the score for the corresponding cell in the table for calculating the R-score is not attributed.

Subsequently, the R$_C$ score should be calculated for the next most serious adverse effect or the most frequent serious adverse effect. Since cough occurred in 37% of patients on enalapril compared to 31% of patients on placebo, and since from the literature it is known that the incidence of cough with ACE-inhibitors occurs in up to 20% of hypertensive patients and leads frequently to discontinuation of therapy (Martindale, 2002), this adverse effect was selected for calculating the R$_C$ score.

An R′ score of 3 is attributed based on an estimated frequency of 'common' (6% excess incidence compared to placebo) and an estimated severity of 'slight' ('temporarily/intermittently incapacitating'). An R′ score of 3 corresponds to an R_C score of 0.

Based on the B-score of 3.5 (conservatively decreased to 3 in order to fit into the TURBO diagram) and an R-score of 3, a T-score of 4 is calculated. This T-score should thus represent the intrinsic benefit–risk balance of enalapril in the treatment of heart failure.

Example: rizatriptan

The properties of rizatriptan in terms of its key safety and efficacy data have been described in the section on the 'Principle of Threes' model. The probability of benefit can be arbitrarily considered as 'frequent', because the pain relief 2 h after treatment was between 67 and 77% with the recommended dose of 10 mg compared to 23 to 40% with placebo. The degree of benefit can be considered as 'slight' which corresponds to a definition that the treated condition (migraine) becomes less frequently incapacitating or incapability is shorter. Although the corresponding B-score is not indicated on the diagram for calculating the B-score, it is logical that a B-score of 3 is assigned. No ancillary benefit is thought to be applicable because rizatriptan only treats the headache associated with migraine.

The medically most serious adverse effect is considered to be myocardial ischemia and infarction, which occur very rarely but are potentially very severe (i.e. life-threatening). According to Table 3.3 this should correspond to an R_0 score of 3. Since the most common adverse effects are dizziness, somnolence and asthaenia/fatigue, in the absence of other serious adverse effects these adverse effects are taken into account for calculating the R_C-score. The incidence of these adverse effects is between 5 and 10% and thus 'common' (if 'common' is defined to be $\geq 1\%$ and $<10\%$), and their estimated severity is 'minor' (defined as some hindrance, but not really incapacitating). It can be assumed from the diagram for calculating the R-score (Table 3.3) that R′ is less than 3 and that therefore $R_C = 0$. The risk factor R which is the sum of R_0 and R_C is thus 3.

According to the TURBO-diagram, a benefit score of 3 and a risk score of 3 correspond to a T-score of 4.

Strengths and weaknesses of the model

Strengths of the model

A merit of this model is that five categories and corresponding definitions for the degree of benefit and for the severity of adverse effects are proposed. The other models allow much less discrimination with regard to these specific parameters.

Another merit of this model is that it tries to consolidate benefit and risk in one score which should represent the intrinsic or absolute benefit–risk balance of a medicine. However, given that this model is in its current form still a draft which needs to be further developed with regard to the definitions for probability of benefit and estimated attributable risk, and with regard to the diagrams for calculating the B-score, the R-score and the T-score, it is difficult to predict whether or not this model could accurately reflect the benefit–risk balance of a medicine.

Weaknesses of the model
This model has the following main disadvantages.

- The model covers essentially only one of the benefit criteria established in Chapter 2 (i.e. 'efficacy versus comparator and its clinical relevance') and one of the risk criteria (i.e. 'incidence, seriousness and duration of specific adverse effects') but ignores all other criteria.

- It is questionable whether the risks of a medicine can be adequately quantified and qualified by taking into account only the medically most serious adverse effect and the next most serious adverse effect (or if there is no next most serious adverse effect, the most frequent adverse effect). For medicines for non-serious diseases and for OTC medicines the overall frequency rather than the seriousness of specific adverse effects might be the issue. In addition, calculating the R-factor requires a subjective decision pertaining to which is the most serious adverse effect, and therefore clear criteria should be provided for this purpose.

- The model further assumes that the R-score associated with the most serious adverse effect (R_0, ranges from 1 to 5) is on average three times more important than the R-score associated with the next most serious adverse effect (R_C, ranges from 0 to 2). It is obvious that for many medicines this is not true.

- The table for calculating the R-score has several deficiencies, i.e. there are no definitions for the frequency categories (CIOMS III definitions should ideally be used for this purpose), it is unclear whether the categories for estimated severity have been validated and their justification is lacking, and most importantly the scores for several cells have not (yet) been attributed.

- The disadvantages of this model with regard to benefit are very similar to the disadvantages for the risk factor, i.e. the categories for quantifying the probability of benefit and the degree of benefit are not well defined and have not been justified or validated.

- The scores for the majority of the cells to calculate the B-score have not been attributed.

- It is unclear what the ancillary benefit should actually represent, i.e. what constitutes an 'ancillary medical property relevant to the indication', and what is meant with an 'ancillary practical property'. This is particularly important since the B_C score can significantly contribute to the B-score, i.e. one or two points to the maximum B-score of 7.

- It is not clarified whether the absolute probability of benefit should be taken into account in the model, or the relative probability of benefit in comparison to the placebo-controlled or active comparator-controlled group if such a group would exist in the pertinent clinical studies. Clear guidance is required in this respect.

- The TURBO diagram which should calculate the T-score based upon the R-score and B-score has not been fully developed. It is logical that a medicine with a maximum risk-factor of 7 and a minimal benefit-factor of 1 should have the lowest T-score, and vice versa that a medicine with a minimal risk-factor of 1 and a maximal benefit-factor of 7 should have the maximum T-score. However, questions can certainly be raised with regard to other T-scores, for example should a medicine with minimal risk and benefit have the same T-score (T = 4) as a medicine with maximal benefit and risk? Also, based on the two above examples, it is questionable if the sensitivity of this model is sufficient. Both medicines have the same T-score, whilst it is generally assumed that ACE-inhibitors have significantly contributed over the last years to prolong the life of patients with congestive heart failure.

- The model has not been validated and its actual use seems to be either very limited or non-existing.

It is acknowledged that balancing the risks and benefits of a medicine and trying to quantify them in one overall score for a given medicine for a given indication is probably the most difficult exercise, and maybe not even possible, in developing a model for benefit–risk assessment. Hence this should be done based upon a clear methodology and eventually be fully validated in order to be applicable in practice.

Finally, the above model for quantifying the risks and benefit of a medicine is merely a framework model that must be further developed. It is questionable whether this model can be used as such, since it has not yet been fully developed and validated. In practice, it seems that its use is very limited at present. However, it is doubtful that even fully developed it would be able to adequately quantify and qualify the benefit–risk profile of a medicine.

The evidence-based benefit and risk model

Background, concept and purpose of the model

Beckmann (1999) examined the benefit–risk profile of medicines from the point of view of the regulatory authorities, which have to decide on approval of new medicines and have to re-evaluate marketed medicines when safety issues arise. He tried to establish a model which maps the current practices of regulatory authorities. In this respect, the key feature in his model is that he takes into account the available evidence for the benefit and risks.

Description of the model

Beckmann (1999) described a model in which the evidence-weighted benefit is balanced against the sum of all evidence weighted risks. In this model, the benefit of a medicine is evaluated separately for each indication, and it is defined as the product of the efficacy in the indication, and the responder rate. According to Beckmann, efficacy can either be evaluated with a 'yes' or 'no' according to a dichotomous qualitative effect (e.g. eradication of *Helicobacter pylori*), in which case the benefit of the effect is clear and will be approximately the same for each patient (but the responder rate will in most cases not be 100%). Alternatively, the evaluated efficacy endpoint of a medicine is quantitatively variable in a continuum of degrees. In this case, a mean value can be given for the degree of the effect around which the efficacy in the treated population spreads. In addition to efficacy and responder rate, a third dimension is established – the evidence for the benefit, or, in more specific terms, the evidence that proves that the benefit really does have the significance that the aforementioned product claims. The reason for adding this third dimension is that regulatory authorities, both during the assessment of a new medicine and during the post-marketing assessment, cannot base their decisions exclusively on established findings, but must act on the basis of plausible assumptions or a well-founded suspicion (e.g. surrogate endpoints instead of hard clinical endpoints in the clinical trials). In this respect, Beckmann mentioned that the evidence depends on the reliability of the data and he described a hierarchy of evidence. This hierarchy moves from high to low as follows: randomized controlled intervention trials – non-randomized controlled intervention trials – controlled observational studies – case series – reported experience from 'authorities' – no data.

The 'evidence-weighted benefit' is thus the product of (1) the efficacy of a medicine in a given indication, (2) the responder rate, and (3) the evidence for the benefit. Beckmann also pictured the evidence-weighted benefit graphically as a cuboid or box (Figure 3.1).

The risk associated with the use of a medicine is presented by the sum of all adverse drug effects possible in a given situation. The dimensions by which the risk of a medicine are evaluated and measured on the basis of adverse drug effects are analogous with those described for benefit. The risk related to a certain type of adverse drug effects is thus defined as the product of its seriousness and the frequency with which it occurs. Beckmann proposed to use the criteria established by the WHO to classify the degree of seriousness of a given adverse drug effect (WHO Collaborating Centre for International Drug Monitoring, 2004). As for the frequency of an adverse drug effect,

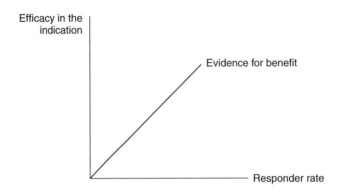

Figure 3.1   'Evidence-weighted benefit' (Reproduced from Beckmann 1999)

according to Beckmann several systems have been used and can be found in product prescribing information. The CIOMS Working Group III has proposed the following classification:

- very common: incidence >10%

- common: incidence 1–10%

- uncommon: incidence 0.1–1%

- rare: incidence 0.01–0.1%

- very rare: <0.01%.

In Germany however a different classification was still in use at the time of publication of this model:

- frequent: incidence >10%

- occasional: incidence 1–10%

- rare: incidence 0.1–1%

- single cases: <0.1%.

The evidence with which a risk can be substantiated has a significant influence on the degree to which the risk argument plays a role in the benefit risk evaluation. For example, despite the fact that randomized, controlled clinical trials are at the top of the hierarchy of sources to demonstrate a given adverse effect, they can only describe and quantify relatively frequent adverse effects due to their limited sample size. On the other hand, for some adverse effects, there can be little available evidence, for example only a theoretical–pharmacological basis, animal data, or poorly documented individual case reports. Therefore, a third dimension is added: the evidence for the risk caused by the adverse effect.

The 'evidence-weighted risk' is thus the product of: (1) the seriousness of the adverse effect; (2) the frequency of the adverse effect; and (3) the evidence for the risk caused by the adverse effect. Similar to the evidence-weighted benefit, the evidence-weighted risk is also graphically represented as a cuboid or box (Figure 3.2). It should finally be noted that each adverse effect observed with a given medicine has its own individual characteristics with regard to the three aforementioned characteristics and thus forms its own box. Assessing the evidence-based risk for each individual adverse effect and calculating the sum of all evidence-based risks is, however, considered to be hardly feasible, and therefore Beckmann argued that in many cases the focus should be on the key adverse effects.

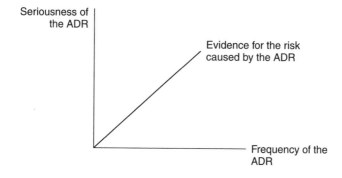

Figure 3.2 'Evidence-weighted risk' (Reproduced from Beckmann 1999)

A new medicine is thus approvable if the evidence-based benefit for the claimed indication outweighs the sum of all evidence-weighted risks. Or, for a marketed product a regulatory procedure might be initiated when it is believed that the sum of all evidence-based risks outweighs the evidence-based benefit.

Beckmann also proposed measures by which a regulatory authority can improve the arguments for a favourable benefit–risk balance of a medicine:

1. improving efficacy: galenics, bioavailability, restriction of indications to persons who react well, changes in therapy regimen (dosing, type of administration)

2. improving the responder rate: non-response as a relative contraindication

3. improving the evidence for benefit: initiation of further studies

4. reducing the seriousness of adverse drug reactions: improvement of pharmaceutical quality, warnings with regard to risk factors (e.g. alcohol), information on adverse effects and first-aid treatment

5. reducing the frequency of adverse effects: inclusion of contraindications, warnings with regard to risk factors (possibly suspension or withdrawal of authorization)

6. improving the evidence for safety: ordering additional studies that could improve the understanding of the risk or refute it.

Finally, Beckmann stated that the concept of 'boxes' for evidence-weighted benefit and evidence-weighted risk should be further elaborated, in particular by developing quantitative scales for each parameter/dimension of benefit and risk description.

Application of the model

There are apparently no publications which describe the benefit–risk profile of a medicine according to this model.

Strengths and weaknesses of the model

Strengths of the model

Beckmann (1999) pointed out that the benefit of a medicine is based on both the level of improvement caused by the medicine, and the responder rate. The third dimension that he added – the evidence for the benefit – is another very important factor which is definitely worth taking into account. As discussed in Chapter 2, the evidence of the clinical benefit might not be absolute, especially during the assessment of a new marketing authorization application. For example, the proof of efficacy might have been based on surrogate endpoints (e.g. bone mineral density instead of fracture incidence data for medicines used to treat osteoporosis, blood cholesterol values instead of incidence of coronary events for medicines used to treat hypercholesterolemia), the efficacy results might not have been fully replicated in all pivotal clinical trials, or the number of patients evaluable for efficacy might be small and/or not fully representative for the normal patient population (Lasagna, 1998). Further evidence of efficacy is usually gathered in additional clinical trials after commercialization of a medicine, and thus the evidence-weighted benefit would correctly become more positive if additional proof of benefit became available. This approach reflects the reality with which regulatory authorities are confronted when they assess medicines. This third dimension can also be considered as an overall criterion that encompasses the benefit criteria established in Chapter 2 (with the exception of 'efficacy versus comparator and its clinical relevance', which is covered in the other two dimensions of the model, and 'anticipated patient compliance in marketed use'):

- design, conduct and statistical adequacy of the trial (for each pivotal trial)
- clinical relevance of the primary endpoints (for each pivotal trial)

- representativeness of the studied population for the population targeted in the label (for each pivotal trial)

- statistical significance of the efficacy results (for each pivotal trial)

- evidence for the efficacy in relevant subgroups (for each pivotal trial)

- confirmation of efficacy by results of non-primary endpoints (for each pivotal trial)

- confirmation of efficacy by results of relevant non-pivotal trials and extensions

- clustering (consistency) of results of the pivotal trials.

On the risk side, Beckmann is equally correct in taking into account not only the seriousness and the frequency of an adverse effect, but also the evidence for the risk caused. As Beckmann pointed out, in clinical studies only relatively frequent adverse effects are detected due to the limited sample size. On the other hand, for adverse effects noted from post-marketing spontaneous reporting, the evidence for causal relationship and the evidence on the incidence might be limited. This third dimension can be considered as an overall criterion that encompasses a number of the risk criteria established in Chapter 2:

- safety in subgroups

- potential for non-demonstrated additional risk due to limitations of clinical trials and/or short market exposure

- potential for non-demonstrated additional risk due to safety issues observed in preclinical safety studies but not in humans

- potential for non-demonstrated additional risk due to safety issues observed with other medicines of the same pharmacological class.

Weaknesses of the model
This model is a framework that needs much further development in order to be applicable in practice. Specifically, the scales need to be developed for each of the three parameters for benefit and risk. In particular, quantifying the 'evidence for the benefit' and the 'evidence for the risk caused by the adverse effect' might turn out to be difficult. It is also doubtful if only the criteria of the WHO should be used to estimate the seriousness of an adverse effect, because the WHO criteria only discriminate between serious and non-serious adverse effects. A more sensitive scale may be

required. Also, additional criteria as identified in Chapter 2 should be taken into consideration to obtain the full picture about the risk side of a medicine:

- overall incidence of adverse effects

- overall incidence of serious adverse effects

- discontinuation rate due to adverse effects

- interactions with other drugs and food

- potential for off-label use leading to safety hazards.

Another major difficulty will be to calculate the sum of all evidence-based risks, which is indeed hardly feasible, as correctly suggested by Beckmann. One option could be to focus only on the key adverse effects, but then clear criteria should be established to identify those key adverse effects.

As with any other models, the most difficult problem will be to develop and validate the scales for benefit and risk in such a way that the balance of both is a true representation of the benefit–risk profile and that the model can correctly distinguish medicines with a negative benefit–risk balance, which should not be approved, from approvable medicines with a favourable benefit–risk balance.

3.3   REVIEW OF MODELS IN SINGLE CLINICAL TRIALS AND FOR SPECIFIC MEDICINES

Background

Apart from the three models discussed above, no model exists which has the capacity to take into account the data from multiple clinical trials and from post-marketing safety data. Several models have however been described which have as their objective to establish a benefit–risk ratio based on the efficacy and safety results of one clinical trial with a given medicine. These models cannot, however, be easily extrapolated to multiple clinical trials and to the data included in a complete marketing authorization application. In addition, most models measure the benefit and risk components based on the individual patient data, and thus require access to those data. Regulatory authorities (in particular in the EU) have, however, no access to the trial database and do not recalculate study results. For these two reasons these models cannot be used within the scope of the current research.

Nevertheless, some of the models might include some interesting features which might be useful in the development of a new model. The models which are most frequently cited in the literature are the model developed by Chuang-Stein called 'Benefit-Less-Risk Analysis in Clinical Trials' (Chuang-Stein, 1994), and the model based on NNT versus numbers needed to harm (NNH) (Mancini and Schulzer, 1999). Because both models include some interesting concepts, in particular with regard to risk calculation and with regard to weighing the benefits and risks, they are discussed hereafter in some detail. Other models are very briefly discussed with the purpose of giving a general overview of the available models, but no attempt is made to review all existing models.

Besides the models which have been established for benefit–risk assessment based on the efficacy and safety results from a single clinical trial, some models have also been developed for specific medicines or therapeutic classes of medicines. Whilst these models cannot be easily extrapolated to other medicines because they are very specific in terms of the measured benefit and risk, some of these models are briefly discussed in order to complete the picture.

Benefit-less-risk analysis in clinical trials

This method discounts the observed benefit of a treatment by the observed risk. This discounting, applied to each individual in a trial, utilizes a method to consolidate the safety data collected in the trial. The collating of the safety information allows the quantitative estimation of the risk experienced by each individual, and therefore enables the construction of a risk-adjusted benefit measure for the same individual.

The approach proposed by Chuang-Stein for risk calculation has three basic assumptions.

1. A set of j classes representative of body functions can be selected to cover all areas of safety concerns for a particular situation under consideration. The total number of classes should be adequate but not overwhelming. An example is to use 10 classes designated as cardiovascular, haematological, gastrointestinal/hepatic, genitourinary/renal, neurological/psychiatric, pulmonary, special senses, metabolic/nutritional, dermatologic, and musculoskeletal.

2. An overall intensity grade k can be determined for each patient within each class j using all the safety information relevant to that class. The intensity grades are set up in such a way that higher grades warrant greater safety concern and the zero grade implies no adverse experience. The total number of intensity grades can vary from class to class. Classes suggesting a more serious safety concern can have a finer intensity grading than the non-serious ones.

3. A weight W_{jk} can be assigned to the kth intensity grade within the jth event class. Higher weights correspond to higher intensity grades and thus represent worse safety outcomes within the class. Furthermore, the approach assumes that the weights can also reflect the relative seriousness of the various intensity grades across different classes.

An individual's total safety score is the sum of the weights assigned to the intensity grades that describe the individual's overall safety experience. The normalized safety score is computed for each individual, which is the ratio between an individual's safety score and the maximum total score, which would represent an individual who experiences side effects of the worst grade in all event classes. This normalized score has a value between 0 and 1 and can be viewed as a summary of risk for an individual.

To adjust the observed benefit by risk, Chuang-Stein proposes to discount the observed benefit by a fraction of the risk summary to obtain a risk-adjusted benefit. Chuang-Stein's approach uses a concept similar to that underlying the adjustment to the life expectancy to obtain the quality-adjusted life expectancy. If we let r_{ti} represent the risk summary for the ith individual in the tth treatment group, and e_{ti} the observed benefit for the same individual, Chuang-Stein proposes to obtain a risk-adjusted benefit as

$$e_{ti}^* = e_{ti} - f \times r_{ti}$$

where f controls the amount of discounting that will take place. The choice of f in the algorithm depends on many factors such as other available treatments and the nature of the disease/symptoms. Since benefit is adjusted for risk by subtracting a multiple of the risk from benefit, the net benefit measure e^*_{ti} was termed 'benefit-less-risk' by Chuang-Stein. She proposes to use this benefit-less-risk for the comparisons between the treatment groups as it were the actual data.

When the efficacy of an intervention is measured on an interval scale, the change in response from its baseline value is typically used to estimate the benefit e_{ti}. When the efficacy is measured by a binary response variable, it is proposed that e_{ti} be 1 if a response is obtained and 0 other-wise. If the response is measured on an ordinal scale and there are numerical values associated with the categories, the appropriate difference in the numeric values will be used for e_{ti}.

This model provides in particular a detailed methodology for assessing the safety data from a clinical trial. It is based on the assumptions that the relative seriousness of adverse effects can be calculated per body system, and that the weights assigned to the intensity grades also reflect the relative seriousness across different body systems. It is however questionable whether it is appropriate to calculate an overall risk score essentially based on body systems instead of individual adverse effects. Even for an individual medicine, it is impractical or even impossible to determine what the relative seriousness is of for instance the cardiovascular adverse effects versus the pulmonary adverse effects. An approach based on the assessment of individual adverse effects would most likely be more accurate.

In addition, many assumptions are required for calculating the net benefit measure e^*_{ti} termed 'benefit-less-risk', such as the intensity grades for each class, the weights assigned to the intensity grades, and the factor f, which controls the fraction of the risk summary that is subtracted from the benefit score. Therefore, a full validation of this model would be required before it could be used accurately in practice.

On the positive side, this model attempts to calculate an overall net benefit score which in theory would allow comparing two different treatments. The concept of the f-factor allows to determine what would be an acceptable risk taking into account the potential benefits of the therapy and the nature of the disease. The overall merit of the model is that it calculates the overall burden due to adverse effects and subtracts this from the benefit, taking into account the nature of the disease and other available treatments, and as such calculates a net benefit score.

Numbers Needed to Treat versus Numbers Needed to Harm

The NNT statistic is potentially a clinically useful measure of treatment effect, conveying both statistical and clinical importance (Smith and Egger, 1994). Its use in the literature and by health authorities seems to be increasing.

Mancini and Schulzer (1999) developed a mathematical model based on the concepts of NNT, which is defined as the reciprocal of the absolute risk reduction due to a given therapy and conveys the effort that must be expended on average to accomplish a single, tangible, and positive outcome in a patient, and NNH, which conveys the treatment effort expended before one patient experiences an adverse treatment-related outcome. They tried to overcome the issues that: (1) NNT conveys the effort required to achieve a positive outcome without distinguishing between the presence or absence of treatment-related adverse events; and (2) NNH conveys harm without accounting for the achievement or lack of achievement of the benefit of therapy. Consequently, a mathematical model was developed to extend the NNT and NNH to represent the effort required to achieve 'unqualified success' (NNT_{US}, treatment success without treatment-induced side effects) and 'unmitigated failure' (NNH_{UF}, lack of treatment success with treatment-induced side effects). NNT_{US} was calculated by adjusting the absolute risk reduction to allow for the probability of not incurring a treatment-related adverse event. NNH_{UF} was similarly calculated by adjusting the absolute risk of incurring a treatment-related adverse event by the probability of not incurring any treatment-related benefit. Mancini and Schulzer concluded that NNT_{US} and NNH_{UF} balance benefit and risk in an objective way and are relevant for making service delivery decisions.

Willan *et al.* developed a similar model by examining how the concept of NNT can be used to improve the presentation of clinical trials data of efficacy and side effects to give clinicians a more clinically meaningful and quantitative measure of benefit–risk trade-offs (Willan *et al.*, 1997). A benefit–risk ratio was established that quantifies for a new therapy how many therapeutic (efficacy) events will be achieved for each adverse event incurred. It was shown how data from a clinical trial with single binary measure of efficacy and a single adverse event of concern can be used to provide point estimates and confidence intervals for the benefit–risk ratio.

An approach to incorporating multiple adverse events into NNT analysis was proposed by Guyatt *et al*. (1999). To take the importance of the relevant adverse events relative to the benefit into account, patients' preference was used by adding the relative utility value into the NNH calculation. However, a limitation of this approach is the availability of utilities, in particular obtaining complex utilities for adverse events given an existing condition (Holden, 2003). Examples of using this method have been described by Holden *et al*. (2003b).

All three models share important disadvantages. It is unclear how these models would account for multiple benefit-variables (e.g. new medicines for rheumatoid arthritis are usually tested using combined primary endpoints such as physician's global assessment of disease activity, patient's global assessment of disease activity, and pain score) (CPMP, 2003b), and, with the exception of the method described by Guyatt *et al*., multiple adverse events of different seriousness. Second, the NNT measure is highly dependent on baseline risk and the duration of treatment as well as the relative risk reduction (Smeeth *et al*., 1999). Therefore, the use of NNT is potentially misleading when used to calculate a benefit–risk ratio based on several studies of different durations and with populations with a different baseline risk. Lastly, these are quantitative mathematical methods that do not incorporate clinical judgement, which is however a key feature of benefit–risk analysis (Holden *et al*., 2003b).

Other models for individual clinical trial results

Shakespeare *et al*. (2001) presented a new concept for the calculation and interpretation of the efficacy results and safety results of a given clinical trial. They proposed to use confidence levels and plotting of clinical significance curves and risk–benefit contours. These curves and contours provide degrees of probability of both the potential benefit of treatment and the detriment due to toxicity. As for benefit, the potential relative benefit (for instance expressed by hazard ratios) is plotted against the corresponding confidence level, which could also be termed 'probability'. Logically, a decrease in confidence is observed with increasing benefit. The same can be done with regard to risk – the potential relative toxicity detriment (in the example included in the article the absolute toxicity detriment is the percentage increased risk to have grade 3 or grade 4 acute toxicity with chemoradiotherapy compared to standard treatment) is plotted against the corresponding confidence level, and provides a clinical significance curve with regard to toxicity. Eventually, the risk–benefit contours, which is a graph that gives a single probability of the benefit and detriment of the new therapy versus the comparator, is established. Assuming that benefit and risk are independent, the risk contour is a product of the two sets of confidence levels. Risk–benefit contours can therefore be defined as a series of curves that join equal levels of confidence (or probability) associated with the risks and benefits of one intervention when compared with another. Thus, each contour (identified with a percentage probability) connects identical probabilities for various risk–benefit scenarios.

This concept is appealing because (1) it is based on clear statistical principles, (2) it allows anyone to make its own conclusions with regard to the probability of benefit and the probability of benefit–risk as an integrated measure, and (3) it is a relatively simple concept. However, it remains to be seen if the safety results of a clinical trial can be expressed for all kind of trials and medicines as the toxicity detriment versus the active control treatment or versus placebo. For many medicines and trials (with the possible exception of anticancer therapy), it is difficult to conclude if for a given patient the test treatment and control treatment are toxic or non-toxic. Nevertheless, the concept proposed by Shakespeare *et al.* is interesting as it integrates the safety and efficacy results of a clinical trial in what they call 'risk–benefit contours'.

Troche *et al.* (2000) developed a patient-specific drug safety-efficacy index that combines objective clinical trial information about dose-related efficacy and toxicity, with subjective perspectives on the trade-off of increased risk for increased efficacy using the probability trade-off technique for patient preferences. Their goal was to allow decision makers to make a more informed choice of medicines and dose levels by developing a tool for combining subjective and objective information about a medicine. Obvious issues with this method which make it not useful within the scope of this research is that patient preferences have to be captured, and that non dose-related adverse effects (e.g. idiosyncratic drug reactions) are not taken into account.

Eriksen and Keller (1993) established an approach for weighing risks and benefits by combining utility functions for human efficacy and toxicity with animal and laboratory toxicity information to develop an overall multi-attribute utility function. They compared this multi-attribute function with the expected utility of several doses of a medicine and argued the value of this approach in drug-dosage selection. This method places too much emphasis on animal and laboratory toxicity data, at the expense of human safety data. It has, however, the merit of relaying some useful concepts used in decision-making analysis, which are further described in Chapter 5.

Models for specific medicines

In this section, three examples of models for benefit–risk assessment of specific medicines or therapeutic classes of medicines are provided. These models apply in general to specific outcome measures used for the subject class of medicines. In case the models are able to take into account multiple studies, it is required that those studies are similar in design. Thus, these models cannot be made easily applicable to other classes of medicines.

Belsey (2001) presented a method which pictures the benefit–risk profile of each of the oral triptans for the treatment of migraine. In this method, the efficacy and safety data from the available clinical trials are pooled for each of the triptans and then plotted by using an *XY* visual analogue graph. Two different methods are used to quantify benefits and risks. The first method uses therapeutic gain, which is defined as the percentage of patients treated with the triptan that is pain free at 2 h minus the percentage of patients treated with placebo that is pain free at 2 h, versus therapeutic penalty, which is defined as the incidence of adverse events in patients treated with the triptan minus the incidence of adverse events in patients treated with placebo. The second method uses NNT versus NNH. Since no single measure exists to express the trade-off between efficacy and tolerability in the management of migraine, the relative performance of each triptan was compared on the visual analogue graph with that of the most commonly prescribed oral triptan which is sumatriptan 100 mg.

Puliyel (2002) described a very simple mathematical model for the benefit–risk assessment of vaccines. In this model (1) the lifetime risk (fraction) of an individual getting the disease multiplied by the fraction of those with disease likely to develop a serious complication, is listed against (2) the fraction of those vaccinated who develop a serious complication attributable to the vaccine multiplied by the fraction of patients protected against the disease by the vaccine. Fraction (1) should be greater than fraction (2) for the vaccine to be used.

Costantino (2001) developed a methodology to perform benefit–risk assessment pertaining to SERMs based on the results of the Breast Cancer Prevention Trial. The method used to assess SERMs includes procedures for estimating the treatment effects for each of the 10 different health endpoints that are potentially affected by therapy with a SERM. To accomplish this, estimates of the expected incidence rate for each of the endpoints are multiplied by the end-point specific risk ratios seen in the Breast Cancer Prevention Trial population.

As described in Chapter 1, Loke *et al.* (2003) developed a benefit–risk analysis of aspirin therapy which allowed quantifying the reduction in cardiovascular events and the increase in gastrointestinal haemorrhage in an individual patient, according to the individual risk profile.

Thompson *et al.* (2003) reviewed the results of the Prostate Cancer Prevention Trial with finasteride, which demonstrated a 24.8% reduction in prostate cancer risk with the administration of finasteride compared to placebo. However, the incidence of high-grade cancers was higher in the finasteride group (6.4%) than in the placebo group (5.1%). Based on the results of the trial, the authors established a matrix of benefits and risks of finasteride administration (Table 3.6). They concluded that the discussion on benefits and risks should include an examination of the 6% absolute prostate cancer risk reduction and 1.3% absolute potential increase in high-grade disease. They added that, just as with almost every other disease prevention intervention, it will be the balance between the benefits and risks, integrated with the patient's own set of priorities and perspectives that will dictate whether finasteride should be employed.

Table 3.6   Matrix of the benefits and risks of finasteride for the prevention of prostate cancer

Benefit/risk	Absolute difference (%)	In favour of:
Prostate cancer diagnosis	6	Finasteride
Genitourinary symptoms and complications	0.3–3.5	Finasteride
Sexual dysfunction or endocrine symptoms	1.7–13.1	Placebo
High-grade cancer diagnosis	1.3	Placebo

A quantitative approach called minimum clinical efficacy (MCE) was first introduced by Djulbegovic and Hozo (1998) as a means of choosing high-dose or low-dose chemotherapy for the adjuvant treatment of breast cancer, and was fine-tuned for general use and applied by Holden *et al.* (2003a, b). MCE of a new treatment is the minimal clinical efficacy needed for it to be worth considering as an alternative treatment after taking into account: (1) the efficacy of the standard treatment; (2) the adverse event profiles associated with the standard treatment and the new treatment; and (3) the risk of disease associated with no treatment. The uniqueness of this approach is that it takes into account not only the benefits and harms of the new and standard treatments, but also the natural characteristics of the disease in the general population, represented by the untreated group. The major weakness of MCE is that its statistical properties are unstudied, and it is therefore unknown whether, for example, confidence intervals for the minimum efficacy can be constructed Holden *et al.* (2003a). In contrast to NNT analysis, MCE has not been widely used in epidemiology.

3.4   CONCLUSION

In this chapter, the three general models for benefit–risk assessment have been reviewed in detail.

1. The 'Principle of Threes' model by Edwards *et al.*, which is most advanced in its development.

2. The evidence-based benefit and risk model by Beckmann, which is a concept model.

3. The TURBO model by Amery, which is a framework model.

Table 3.7 summarizes these three models and their attributes.

Table 3.7   Summary of the attributes in the existing models for benefit–risk assessment

	'Principle of Threes' grading system	TURBO model	Evidence-based benefit and risk model
Benefit attributes			
Seriousness of improvement	✓	✓	✓
Duration of improvement	✓		
Probability of improvement	✓	✓	✓
Evidence for the benefit			✓
Risk attributes			
Seriousness of the adverse effects	✓	✓	✓
Duration of the adverse effects	✓		
Incidence of the adverse effects	✓	✓	✓
Evidence for the risk			✓
Disease attributes			
Seriousness	✓		
Duration	✓		
Incidence	✓		

With regard to these general models, the following can be concluded.

- Few models exist to balance the benefit–risk profile of medicines.

- Many criteria used in the existing models are not well defined with regard to the type, quality and relative importance of the data to be taken into account (e.g. which clinical studies should be used for the benefit criteria? Which adverse effects should be taken into account?), and the scores to be attributed.

- There is a significant gap between the list of benefit and risk criteria identified in Chapter 2 as being relevant for a model, and the few criteria incorporated in these models, in particular in the 'Principle of Threes' grading system and in the TURBO model. Table 3.8 compares the list of criteria identified in Chapter 2 with the three models.

- The models are not very sophisticated and allow only a very crude benefit–risk assessment.

- Although there are some important flaws in some of the models, there are also some merits and interesting concepts that have been applied, e.g. the evidence for the benefit and risk considered by Beckmann.

Table 3.8 Application of the benefit and risk criteria to the three models

	'Principle of Threes' grading system	TURBO model	Evidence-based benefit and risk model
Benefit criteria			
Efficacy versus comparator and its clinical relevance (for each pivotal trial)	√	√	√
Design, conduct and statistical adequacy of the trial (for each pivotal trial)			√[a]
Clinical relevance of the primary endpoints (for each pivotal trial)			√[a]
Representativeness of the studied population for the population targeted in the label (for each pivotal trial)			√[a]
Statistical significance of the efficacy results (for each pivotal trial)			√[a]
Evidence for the efficacy in relevant subgroups (for each pivotal trial)			√[a]
Efficacy as per the results of the non-primary endpoints (for each pivotal trial)			√[a]
Efficacy as per the results of the relevant non-pivotal trials and extensions			√[a]
Anticipated patient compliance in market use			
Clustering (consistency) of results of the pivotal trials			√[a]
Risk criteria			
Overall incidence of adverse effects			
Overall incidence of serious adverse effects			
Discontinuation rate due to adverse effects			
Incidence, seriousness, duration and reversibility of specific adverse effects	√	√	√
Safety in subgroups			√[a]
Interactions with other drugs and food			
Potential for off-label use leading to safety hazards			
Potential for non-demonstrated additional risk due to limitations of clinical trials and/or length of patient exposure			√[a]
Potential for non-demonstrated additional risk due to safety issues observed in preclinical safety studies but not in humans			√[a]
Potential for non-demonstrated additional risk due to safety issues observed with other medicines of the same pharmacological class			√[a]

[a] Implied in general 'evidence for benefit–risk' criterion.

- None of the models has been validated nor is broadly used in practice. The practical experience obtained by testing the applicability of the 'Principle of Threes' model and the TURBO model confirmed the important flaws of both models which would most likely prevent providing accurate and reproducible results. Their use at present would therefore be premature.

- However, according to some experts in the field with who these models were discussed, the models are helpful to streamline the thoughts on benefit–risk assessment and they contribute conceptually to improve decision-making by regulatory authorities on medicines.

Several models exist which have as their objective either to establish a benefit–risk ratio based on one clinical trial with a given medicine, or to establish a benefit–risk ratio for a specific medicine or therapeutic class of medicines. Whilst some of these models include some interesting features, none of them is able to either encompass the totality of safety and efficacy data from multiple clinical trials and from spontaneous adverse event reporting for a given medicine, or to be easily extrapolated to other classes of medicines.

Finally, no validated, well-accepted models seem to exist that have the appropriate degree of sophistication. A number of models have been described in the literature, some of which are useful to a certain degree, but it is clear that none of the models could serve for further development. This confirms the hypothesis that more research is needed on models for benefit–risk assessment, and that hence it is worthwhile to attempt to develop a new better defined model with sound measurement properties.

3.5 NEWER MODELS

New models as well as variations and applications of existing models continue to be published. A recent OHE Briefing (Appendix 2) reviewed most of these models. In general, these newer models have similar weaknesses as the older models discussed above, which impedes their wider application.

- 'A multiattribute model for evaluating the benefit–risk profiles of treatment alternatives' (Felli *et al.*, 2008).

- 'Update on the methods of the US Preventive Services Task Force: estimating certainty and magnitude of net benefit' (Sawaya *et al.*, 2007).

- 'Application of a unique scoring system for numerical determination of a benefit risk ratio in clinical trials' (Pearce *et al.*, 2008).

- 'Advances in risk benefit evaluation using probabilistic simulation methods: an application to the prophylaxis of deep vein thrombosis' (Lynd and O'Brien, 2004).

- 'Current assessment of risk-benefit by regulators: is it time to introduce decision analysis?' (Hughes *et al.*, 2007).

- 'Joint distribution approaches to simultaneously quantifying benefit and risk' (Shaffer and Watterberg, 2006).

- 'Net Efficacy adjusted for risk (NEAR): a simple procedure for measuring risk:benefit balance' (Boada *et al.*, 2008).

- 'Global benefit–risk assessment in designing clinical trials and some statistical considerations of the method' (Pritchett and Tamura, 2007).

- 'Simultaneous comparison of multiple treatments: combining direct and indirect evidence' (Caldwell *et al.*, 2005).

- 'Relative risks and confidence intervals were easily computed indirectly from multivariable logistic regression' (Localio *et al.*, 2007).

CHAPTER 4

Defining a Systematic Approach to Decision Making

4.1 INTRODUCTION

One of the most important if not the most important use of benefit–risk assessment pertains to the approval of new medicines by regulatory authorities and the subsequent review of these products during their life-cycle when new safety and/or efficacy data become available. These decisions by regulatory authorities may have a major impact on public health, in particular the approval of innovative medicines for serious diseases, the withdrawal of marketed medicines because of major safety issues, and significant label changes which either restrict or expand the use of a medicine. Although a limited number of methods and models for benefit–risk assessment exist, most of them have been proposed for the re-assessment of marketed medicines when a new safety issue arises. However, it seems that these methods are not widely used by regulatory authorities. Thus, it is plausible to ask whether the use of such methods would aid decision making by regulatory authorities and benefit the interactions with the other key stakeholders such as pharmaceutical companies, prescribers and patients.

Based on the review conducted in Chapter 1, it appears that, overall, limited research has been conducted in the area of methods and models for benefit–risk assessment pertaining to the approval of new medicines and the re-assessment of marketed medicines. The first part of this book therefore focused on evaluating the current practices and methods for benefit–risk assessment. Based on that review, a model for benefit–risk assessment will be developed in order to determine whether such a model can be used as a valid tool for the assessment of new medicines and the re-assessment of marketed medicines.

Unlike the existing models, it is conceptualized that the new model will utilize all available efficacy and safety data. To this effect it is envisaged that due to its

Benefit-Risk Appraisal of Medicines   Filip Mussen, Sam Salek, Stuart Walker
© 2009 John Wiley & Sons, Ltd

comprehensive nature, validity and sophistication, such a model will be welcomed by the stakeholders and prove to be of significant value in practice. Nevertheless, a number of challenges are anticipated in finding and developing the best possible model (Evans, 2008), most of which pertain to the fact that the benefit–risk balance of a medicine is essentially a value judgement.

- It remains to be seen whether it is possible to adequately judge and compare in a model apples (benefits) and pears (risks) and to decide whether the apples outweigh the pears or vice-versa;

- Whilst a model should most likely work in situations where a medicine has major benefits and minimal risks, or minimal benefits with some major risks, it is unknown whether a model will be of significant value and sensitive enough for more subtle comparisons of benefits and risks.

4.2   OBJECTIVES AND FEATURES OF THE IDEAL MODEL FOR BENEFIT–RISK ASSESSMENT

Based on the literature review and on the general objective established in Chapter 1 to determine if a model for benefit–risk assessment can be used as a valid tool for the assessment of new medicines and the re-assessment of marketed medicines, a number of specific objectives and basic features of an ideal model are outlined. Hence, the review of the existing models and the development of a new model has been conducted keeping the following basic prerequisites in mind.

- In general, a model should match the current practices of regulatory authorities for benefit–risk assessment, which are essentially embedded in the pharmaceutical regulations of the country/region, in order to ensure that the model can be used within the scope of those practices.

- Specifically, a model should be able to take into account the data in a marketing authorization application and the scientific data otherwise available to regulatory agencies. As reviewed in Chapter 2, specific requirements exist with regard to the content of marketing authorization applications, which contain in general data on quality, pre-clinical safety and pharmacology, safety and efficacy data from clinical trials, and post-approval safety data from commercial use if available. Cost and health economic data are not considered by regulatory authorities in Europe and the United States within the scope of the approval process of new medicines or the re-assessment of existing medicines. A model should therefore not take cost factors into account.

- A model should not require additional analyses or re-analyses of source clinical data (safety and efficacy), or additional clinical meta-analyses. Such analyses are usually very complex and would require access to the source data, which regulatory authorities in Europe do not have. Furthermore, performing additional analyses on clinical data is not within the remit of most regulatory authorities.

- As outlined in the objectives of this book, it should be possible to use the same model both during the initial registration process of new medicines, and during the post-approval re-assessment of existing medicines. *A priori*, there is no reason to use a different model at different stages in the life-cycle of a medicine. Moreover, in Chapter 1 it was described that the benefit–risk balance is dynamic and evolves over time. Therefore, it would be of value that a model could measure how the benefit–risk balance evolves.

- A model should be applicable to all kinds of medicines, including vaccines and non-prescription medicines. It may be relatively simple to develop a model for life-saving products, where essentially the mortality benefit must be weighted against the serious adverse effects. However, a universal model will most likely require the incorporation of additional criteria and therefore require a more sophisticated and flexible approach.

- A model should be considered as a tool for regulatory authorities and pharmaceutical industry for assessing the benefit–risk profile of medicines. It does not substitute for making the decision whether the benefits outweigh the risks or vice-versa, but it is an aid for making those decisions. In this respect, a model can make benefit–risk assessments more explicit and transparent, and it can enhance the consistency and objectivity of benefit–risk decisions.

- It should be possible to validate a model, as will be discussed in a next section of this chapter.

4.3 THE USE OF DECISION-ANALYSIS TECHNIQUES FOR THE DEVELOPMENT OF THE NEW MODEL

Decision analysis: scope and process

In this chapter, decision-analysis techniques will be used for the construction of the new model for benefit–risk assessment. The new model will specifically apply multi-criteria decision analysis; this is also called multi-attribute decision analysis. There are a number of reasons why decision analysis techniques and in particular multi-criteria decision analysis is considered to be the best possible basis for a model for benefit–risk assessment. These reasons will be discussed in Chapter 5. In this section however a general overview will be provided on decision analysis and its main features, and on multi-criteria decision analysis including its different schools of thought.

In general, applying decision analysis techniques can lead to better decisions. According to Clemen (1996), there are four basic sources of difficulty with decisions, and a decision analysis approach can help a decision-maker with all four.

1. A decision can be hard because of its complexity. It is sometimes nearly impossible for a decision maker to keep all the issues in mind at one time. Decision analysis provides effective methods for organizing a complex problem into a structure that can be analysed.

2. A decision can be difficult because of the inherent uncertainty in the situation. A decision-analysis approach can help in identifying important sources of uncertainty and representing that uncertainty in a systematic and useful way.

3. A decision maker may be interested in working toward multiple objectives, but progress in one direction may impede progress in others. Decision analysis provides both a framework and specific tools for trading off benefits in one area against issues in another.

4. A problem may be difficult if different perspectives lead to different conclusions. This source of difficulty is particularly pertinent when more than one person is involved in making the decision. Different individuals may look at the problem from different perspectives, or they may disagree on the uncertainty or value of the various outcomes. The use of decision analysis can help to overcome these differences.

Thus, decision analysis is intended to help people deal with difficult decisions, and it allows people to make effective decisions more consistently. Figure 4.1 shows a general flowchart for the decision analysis process. The first step is to identify the decision situation or context and understand the objectives. This has essentially been accomplished in Chapter 1. In addition, in Chapter 3 the current models and practices for benefit–risk assessment have been reviewed, the objective being to better understand the context of the decision. The second step is to identify alternatives, which in the case of benefit–risk assessment is rather straightforward compared to many other problems for which decision analysis is used. The alternatives in the case of benefit–risk assessment of new medicines are either to approve the commercialization of the medicine under discussion, or to approve it but with restrictions to its use in the product label, or not to allow the medicine on the market. The alternatives for existing

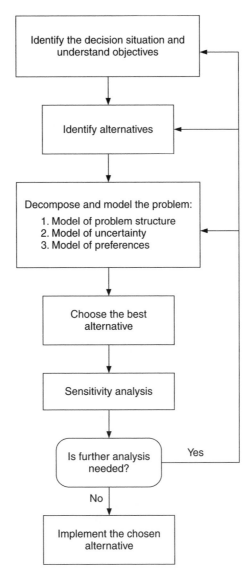

Figure 4.1 Decision-analysis process flowchart (Reproduced from Clemen 1996) © Duxbury Press

medicines are either to maintain the medicine on the market with or without label changes, or not to allow the medicine on the market any longer.

The next two steps are critical in decision analysis. First, decomposing the problem into smaller and more manageable pieces facilitates understanding its structure and measuring uncertainty and value. This was done in detail in Chapter 2, in which all relevant benefit and risk criteria were identified and described. Next, the problem will be modelled. Models can be used in several ways. Influence diagrams or decision trees create a representation or model of the decision problem. Probability can be used to build models of the uncertainty inherent in the problem. Utility functions model the way in which decision makers value different outcomes (preferences) and trade-off competing objectives. This latter approach will be used in Chapter 5 in which a model for benefit–risk assessment based on multi-criteria decision analysis will be constructed. Since these models are mathematical, a key advantage is that the mathematical representation of a decision can be subjected to analysis, which can indicate a 'preferred' alternative. Once a model has been built, sensitivity analysis is performed. Such analysis answers 'what if' questions. By making small changes in one or more aspects of the model, it can be analysed whether the optimal decision changes. If so, the decision is sensitive to these small changes, and those aspects to which the decision is sensitive should subsequently be reconsidered more carefully. The decision maker may return to the identification of the problem, refine the definition of objectives or include new objectives, identify new alternatives, change the structure of the model, or refine the model of uncertainty and preferences. The term 'decision-analysis cycle' best describes the overall process, which may go through several iterations before a satisfactory solution is found.

Before further describing the different decision analysis techniques and models, it is important to define 'values' and 'objectives'. In a general sense 'values' are things that matter to you (Clemen, 1996). For example, a scientist may be interested in resolving a specific scientific question. An 'objective' is a specific thing that you want to achieve. An individual's objectives taken together make up his or her values. They define what is important to that person in making a decision. In the case of the scientist, he or she may want to find an answer to the scientific question in order to gain prestige in the scientific community, which in turn may lead to a higher salary and more research support.

Clemen (1996) divides decision analysis into three main topics, which are modelling decisions, modelling uncertainty, and modelling preferences. Modelling or structuring decisions usually happens by using influence diagrams or decision trees. Both are graphical representations of decision situations which structure decisions and alter-natives, uncertain events and outcomes, and consequences, and which specify how these elements are interrelated. Modelling uncertainty in decision problems is done through the use of probability. Ways to use probability are subjective probability (which recognize that subjective judgements play a central role in decision analysis), theoretical probability models, data-based models, and simulations (Monte Carlo simulation). Modelling preferences pertains to the development of a mathematical representation of a decision-maker's preferences, including the identification of desir-able objectives and trade-offs between conflicting objectives. As trading-off risk and expected value is a fundamental issue, there are several methods to model a decision-maker's attitude toward risk. Furthermore, there are other models for dealing with multiple objectives, in particular multi-attribute decision analysis (also called multi-criteria decision analysis or MCDA), which is a mathematical model that reflects subjective judgements of relative importance among competing objectives.

Multi-criteria decision analysis

According to Belton and Stewart, MCDA is an umbrella term to describe a collection of formal approaches which seek to take explicit account of multiple criteria in helping individuals or groups explore decisions that matter (Belton and Stewart, 2002). Decisions matter when the level of conflict between criteria, or of conflict between different stakeholders regarding what criteria are relevant and the importance of the different criteria, assumes such proportions that intuitive 'gut-feel' decision-making is not satisfactory. MCDA is both an approach and a set of techniques, and has as a goal to provide an overall ordering of options, from the most preferred to the least preferred option (Department for Transport, Local Government and the Regions, 2001). The options may differ in the extent to which they achieve several objectives, and some conflict or trade-off is usually evident amongst the objectives. The first complete exposition of MCDA was given in 1976 by Keeney and Raiffa, who extended decision theory such as decision trees to accommodate multi-attributed consequences.

There are three key phases of the MCDA process: (1) problem identification and structuring; (2) model building and use, which includes the development of formal models of decision-maker preferences, value trade-offs and goals; and (3) development of action plans. The models that have been developed to represent preferences in the context of multi-criteria problems can be classified into three broad categories or schools of thought (Belton and Stewart, 2002.

1. Value measurement models, in which numerical scores are constructed to represent the degree to which one decision option may be preferred to another. Such scores are developed initially for each individual criterion, and are then synthesized and aggregated into higher level preference models.

2. Goal, aspiration or reference level models, in which desirable or satisfactory levels of achievement are established for each of the criteria. The process then seeks to discover options which are closest to achieving these desirable goals.

3. Outranking models, in which alternative courses of action are compared pair-wise, initially in terms of each criterion, in order to identify the extent to which a preference for one over the other can be asserted. In aggregating such preference information across all relevant criteria, the model seeks to establish the strength of evidence favouring selection of one alternative over another.

Further details on these models and how they will be considered for developing the new model for benefit–risk assessment of medicines will be provided in Chapter 5.

According to Belton and Stewart, MCDA has the following features and advantages:

- MCDA takes explicit account of multiple, conflicting criteria

- MCDA helps to structure the problem

- the principal aim of MCDA is to help decision makers learn about the problem, about their own and others values and judgements, and through organization, synthesis and appropriate presentation of information to guide them in identifying a preferred course of action

- MCDA serves to complement and to challenge intuition, but it does not seek to replace intuitive judgement or experience

- MCDA leads to better considered, justifiable and explainable decisions, and it provides an audit trail for a decision

- the most useful approaches of MCDA are conceptually simple and transparent.

The application of MCDA methods generally needs to be supported by appropriate computer software. A number of MCDA software packages are commercially available. The software that is used in Chapter 5 is Hiview 3, from Catalyze Ltd (Winchester, UK). It was developed in association with Enterprise LSE, which was set up by the London School of Economics and Political Science (LSE) to enable and facilitate commercial application of its expertise and intellectual resources.

Relevance and applicability of the model

In 1998, the Council for International Organizations of Medical Sciences (CIOMS) stated that:

> It is a frustrating aspect of benefit–risk evaluation that there is no defined and tested algorithm or summary metric that combines benefit and risk data and that might permit straightforward quantitative comparisons of different treatment options, which in turn might aid in decision making (CIOMS, 1998).

Benefit–risk analysis, despite consuming substantial resources of drug companies, academics and regulators, remains today a concept that is paradoxically and primarily undefined (Holden, 2003). On the other hand, both the FDA and the European regulatory authorities are increasingly requesting benefit–risk analyses of medicines (Holden *et al.*, 2003a). However, such appeals are not accompanied by suggested methods to be used in these analyses, leading to speculation and presumption, and, ultimately, inconsistent or dissimilar investigations. Thus, there is undoubtedly room for a validated model for benefit–risk assessment to be used as a common tool by the regulatory authorities and pharmaceutical companies.

The MCDA-based model is relatively easy to understand and use by people who are not familiar with decision-analysis techniques, which allows focusing on the scientific data and the scores and weights to be derived from those data, instead of on the model itself. The model has also the potential to be superior to the existing practices and methods, such as the current *ad-hoc* benefit–risk assessments or the 'Principle of Threes' and TURBO models. Both within the scope of the initial assessment of new medicines as well as the re-assessment of marketed medicines, the model can make benefit–risk assessments more explicit and transparent, and it can enhance the consistency and objectivity of benefit–risk decisions and thus their overall quality. In addition, the model provides for a common platform for benefit–risk discussions between regulatory authorities and the pharmaceutical companies, which both have a somewhat different focus (i.e. regulatory authorities tend to focus more on risks than on benefits because of their mandate to protect the public health, whilst the reverse may be true for pharmaceutical companies). Another advantage of the model is that it may help the regulatory authorities in publicly expressing the full picture of the evidence and the uncertainties regarding the risks of a medicine in a challenging social climate which is increasingly intolerant of risk and which has created a tendency to seek absolute safety and security (The Uppsala Monitoring Centre, 2002b).

It is of value to consider the potential of an improved quality of benefit–risk decisions within the context of the quality of decisions in general. The quality of decisions has been the subject of significant research. It can be measured, for example with a so-called decision quality spider diagram (Matheson and Matheson, 1998). The spider diagram helps to rate a decision on each of the six dimensions defined by Matheson and Matheson, which together summarize the quality of a decision (Figure 4.2). One hundred per cent is the point at which additional effort to improve this dimension would not be worth the cost. Table 4.1 reviews how each of these dimensions is covered in the different steps of the benefit–risk assessment model, as defined in Chapter 5. With the exception of the sixth dimension (i.e. commitment to action), all dimensions are appropriately included in the benefit–risk assessment model. It is therefore very likely that this model, based on its benchmarking against an instrument which measures the quality of decisions in general, will enhance the quality of the benefit–risk decisions.

The voluntary withdrawal by Merck & Co. of Vioxx (rofecoxib), its blockbuster COX-2 inhibitor because of an excess risk of myocardial infarctions and stroke in the APPROVe trial, only increased the pressure on regulatory authorities and

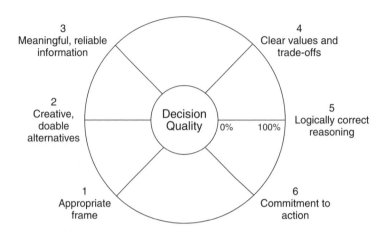

Figure 4.2   Decision quality spider diagram

Table 4.1   Coverage of the dimensions of the spider diagram in the benefit–risk model

Dimensions in the decision quality spider diagram	Corresponding step in the benefit–risk assessment model
1. *Appropriate frame*: the correct background, setting and context for a decision	Step 1: establishment of the decision context (identification of the indication, the dosage, etc.)
2. *Creative, doable alternatives*	Step 2: identification of the options to be appraised (the medicine being assessed and the comparators)
3. *Meaningful, reliable information*	Steps 3: identification of the benefit and risk criteria and organization in a value tree
	Step 4: assessment of the performance of each option against the criteria
	Both steps include sub-steps for the identification of the relevant data including the pivotal and non-pivotal trials and the safety dataset
4. *Clear values and trade-offs*: establishing criteria for measuring the value of alternatives and making rational trade-offs among them	Step 3: identification of the benefit and risk criteria and organization in a value tree
	Step 4: assessment of the performance of each option against the criteria (this is the scoring of the options on the criteria)
5. *Logically correct reasoning*: requires bringing together the inputs of the previous dimensions, usually in a model, to determine which alternatives create the most value	Step 5: assignment of a weight to each criterion
	Step 6: calculation of the weighted scores at each level and calculation of the overall weighted scores
6. *Commitment to action*	None

pharmaceutical companies for making the best possible benefit–risk assessments (Vioxx: an unequal partnership between safety and efficacy, 2004). As a consequence of this dramatic withdrawal, there is a call to regulatory authorities to re-assess the safety and efficacy thresholds required for the licensing of new medicines. Although it is recognized that this is an immensely complicated equation involving, among other factors, the nature of the condition being treated, the therapeutic strategies already available, and the perceived benefit-to-risk hazard profile of the new treatment, the current data requirements and processes for allowing new medicines on the market are being questioned (Vioxx: an unequal partnership between safety and efficacy, 2004). The MCDA-based model could contribute to improving these processes. With respect to the Vioxx withdrawal, the use of the model could make the uncertainty with regard to the absence or insufficiency of data (usually at the time of the initial approval) explicit and could moreover quantify it. Specifically, the three risk criteria 'potential for non-demonstrated additional risk due to limitations of clinical trials and/or length of patient exposure', 'potential for non-demonstrated additional risk due to safety issues observed in pre-clinical safety studies but not in humans', and 'potential for non-demonstrated additional risk due to safety issues observed with other medicines of the same pharma-cological class' (which may now be an important factor for the other COX-2 inhibitors), may capture this uncertainty into the benefit–risk equation.

Development and Application of a Benefit–Risk Assessment Model Based on Multi-Criteria Decision Analysis

5.1 INTRODUCTION

In this chapter, a new model for the benefit–risk assessment of medicines will be described in detail. The model will incorporate as much as possible the findings and prerequisites established in the previous chapters. In this respect, the overall goal of developing the new model is that it should be an improvement when compared to the current methods and practices for benefit–risk assessment. The model will be based on MCDA techniques, which will be described in detail in this chapter, and the rationale and strengths of using MCDA will be demonstrated. The data from an existing medicine (i.e. rizatriptan, for the treatment of migraine) will be used to illustrate the applicability of the new model.

5.2 CONCEPTUALIZATION OF THE NEW MODEL

In Chapter 4, seven prerequisites for a benefit–risk assessment model were defined. Hereafter these prerequisites are consolidated with the proposed benefit and risk criteria described in Chapter 2 and the lessons learned from the review of the current methods and models in Chapter 3. In terms of these prerequisites, a model should do the following.

Benefit-Risk Appraisal of Medicines   Filip Mussen, Sam Salek, Stuart Walker
© 2009 John Wiley & Sons, Ltd

1. Match the current practices of regulatory authorities for benefit–risk assessment.

2. Take into account the efficacy and safety data in a marketing authorization application and the scientific data otherwise available to regulatory agencies. In this respect, 10 efficacy criteria and 10 safety criteria were identified in Chapter 2 based on the ICH, EU and US guidelines. Since these criteria are, in principle, relevant for any kind of medicine, they should be incorporated in any new model.

3. Not require additional analyses or re-analyses of source clinical data (safety and efficacy), or additional meta-analyses. Such analyses are usually very complex and would require access to the source data, which regulatory authorities in Europe and in a number of other countries do not have. Furthermore, performing additional analyses on clinical data is not within the remit of most regulatory authorities, perhaps with the exception of the FDA.

4. Be used both during the initial registration process of new medicines, and during the post-approval re-assessment of existing medicines. *A priori*, there is no reason to use a different model at different stages in the life cycle of a medicine.

5. Be applicable to all categories of medicines, including vaccines and non-prescription medicines. It may be relatively simple to develop a model just for life-saving products, where essentially the mortality benefit must be weighted against the serious adverse effects. However, a universal model will require the incorporation of more criteria and therefore require a more sophisticated and flexible approach than the approach applied to the three models described in Chapter 3 (i.e. the 'Principle of Threes' grading system, the TURBO model, and the evidence-based benefit and risk model).

6. Be considered as a tool for regulatory authorities and pharmaceutical industry for assessing the benefit–risk profile of medicines. It does not substitute for making the decision whether the benefits outweigh the risks or vice-versa, but it is an aid for making such decisions. In this respect, a model can make benefit–risk assessments more explicit and transparent, and it can enhance the consistency and objectivity of benefit–risk decisions.

7. Withstand validity testing establishing whether the model measures what it purports to measure.

5.3   REASONS FOR USING DECISION ANALYSIS TECHNIQUES IN THE NEW MODEL

As mentioned in Chapter 1, benefit and risk are fundamentally evaluative terms, which contain value judgements that, in principle, cannot be made scientifically (Veatch, 1993). Conducting a benefit–risk assessment requires superimposing evaluative judgements on the scientific facts, such as the available efficacy and safety data. Whilst preclinical and clinical research activity is fundamentally 'truth-driven', with researchers seeking to minimize contamination of the facts by values, policy-making within the scope of benefit–risk assessments is fundamentally decision-driven (Dowie, 1996b). It requires somehow the integration of technical judgements with value judgements. Consequently, a pure mathematical method for benefit–risk assessment is not appropriate. Although mathematical methods have been applied to individual clinical trial results and to specific medicines, as described in Chapter 3, they are not suitable for making value judgements. Instead, Waller and Evans (2003) and Cohen and Neumann (2007) advocated the use of a formal decision-making process involving decision-analysis as a robust method for benefit–risk assessment, which increases transparency, makes reasoning explicit and identifies the limitations of the evidence and uncertainty.

Several other authors have promoted the use of decision-analysis techniques for medical decision-making. According to Lilford *et al.* (1998), the great strength of decision analysis is that it is based not just on probabilities but also on the value placed on various outcomes. It therefore represents a method for synthesizing both medical facts and human values, which together determine the best course of action. Moreover, decision analysis is very useful to integrate the outcomes and the different values attributed to those outcomes from more than one study. According to Dowie (1996a) the primary virtue of analysis-based medical decision making is that it makes explicit, on the one hand, the uncertainties and evidential gaps that science has not removed by way of clinical trials or a less robust method, and, on the other hand, the value differences and conflicts. Furthermore, decision analysis provides the comprehensive framework that identifies the several inputs needed for a decision, and shows how the diverse elements can be systematically and transparently integrated into a choice. It provides the map and the language necessary for the different stakeholders to discuss the different options with regard to the medical decision to be taken. Lilford and Braunholtz (1996) state that decision analysis can be used to trade off the best available estimates of benefit and harm, and they suggest using Bayesian statistics for this purpose. Irrespective of the decision analysis method applied, the limitations of intuitive reasoning and the superiority of actuarial methods over intuitive reasoning in medical decision making are demonstrated in a large amount of empirical literature (Dawes *et al.*, 1989).

5.4   THE USE OF MCDA IN THE NEW MODEL

Reasons for using MCDA

Many decision analysis techniques exist, and an overview of the most important decision analysis approaches was provided in Chapter 4. MCDA is a method of looking at complex problems that are usually characterized by any mixture of monetary and non-monetary objectives, of breaking the problem into more manageable pieces to allow data and judgements to be brought to bear on the pieces, and then of reassembling the pieces to present a coherent overall picture to decision makers (Department for Transport, Local Government and the Regions, 2000). The purpose is to serve as an aid to thinking and decision making, but not to take the decision. As a set of techniques, MCDA provides different ways of disaggregating a complex problem, of measuring the extent to which options achieve objectives, of weighting the objectives, and of reassembling the pieces.

The main reason why the use of MCDA is appropriate and preferable for developing a new model for benefit–risk assessment is that it allows the balancing of multiple criteria. The benefit–risk assessment of medicines is characterized by: (1) the need for taking multiple benefit and risk criteria into account; (2) the fact that the evidence and the potential uncertainty because of the incompleteness of the evidence should be considered (Beckmann, 1999); and (3) the need for making trade-offs of the benefits against the risks, and MCDA allows all of this. In this respect, it should be noted that Troche *et al.* (2000) proposed the use of multi-attribute utility theory functions, which is a technique based on MCDA, during drug development. In addition, Eriksen and Keller (1993) developed and applied such a function. Both applications were briefly described in chapters one and three, respectively. Thus, there are some precedents for the use of MCDA-based techniques for assessing the efficacy and safety data of medicines, although the scope and objectives were different.

Sources on MCDA used to develop the model

The following sources of information and expertise on MCDA were used for the development of the new model for benefit–risk assessment:

- the book *Multiple Criteria Decision Analysis, An Integrated Approach* (Belton and Stewart, 2002), which describes the different methods and schools of MCDA in detail

- the DTLR multi-criteria analysis manual (Department for Transport, Local Government and the Regions, 2000), which provides practical examples of the application of MCDA

- the book *Making Hard Decisions – An Introduction to Decision Analysis* (Clemen, 1996), which puts MCDA in a broader perspective

- advice from an expert in decision analysis (L. Phillips).

Stages of MCDA

There are three key phases of the MCDA process: (1) problem identification and structuring: (2) model building and use: and (3) development of action plans (Belton and Stewart, 2002). More specifically, a detailed step-wise methodology which dissects the first two key phases of the MCDA process has been described (Department for Transport, Local Government and the Regions, 2000). This methodology will be applied as such in the next section for the development of the new model. It can be summarized as follows.

1. Establish the decision context.

2. Identify the options to be appraised.

3. Identify objectives and criteria.

    3.1. Identify criteria for assessing the consequences for each option.

    3.2. Organize the criteria by clustering them under high-level and lower-level objectives in the hierarchy.

4. Assess the expected performance of each option against the criteria ('scoring').

    4.1. Describe the consequences of each option.

    4.2. Score the options on the criteria.

    4.3. Check the consistency of the scores on each criterion.

5. Assign weights for each criterion to reflect their relative importance to the decision.

6. Calculate weighted scores at each level in the hierarchy and calculate overall weighted scores.

7. Examine the result and conduct sensitivity analysis.

5.5   DEVELOPMENT OF THE NEW MODEL

Overview

A schematic overview of the development of the model is presented in Table 5.1. The construction of the model consists of seven steps, and each step is discussed in detail in

Table 5.1   Schematic overview of the development of the benefit–risk assessment model

Step 1	*Establishment of the decision context*
	Identification of the indication, the dosage for that indication, the contraindications, and the other critical safety wording in the proposed product label of the subject medicine
Step 2	*Identification of the options to be appraised*
	(1) the medicine being assessed (2) the comparators (active comparator and/or placebo) used in the pivotal clinical trials
Step 3	*Identification of the benefit and risk criteria and organization in a value tree*
	(1) identification of the pivotal clinical trials and their primary endpoints (2) drawing the value tree as shown in Figure 5.1
Step 4	*Assessment of the performance of each option against the criteria*
	(1) identification of the relevant data including the non-pivotal trials and extension studies, and the safety dataset (2) construction of the scale for each criterion (partial value functions for selected criteria, direct rating for the other criteria), and scoring of each option on each criterion (3) checking of the consistency of the scores on each criterion
Step 5	*Assignment of a weight to each criterion using swing-weighting*
	(1) assignment of the relative weights to the bottom-level benefit criteria under each pivotal trial and under the 'other benefit criteria' (2) assignment of the relative weights of the pivotal trials and the 'other benefit criteria', taking into account the trial confidence criteria (bottom-up approach) (3) assignment of the relative weights to the risk criteria (4) assignment of the relative weights to the benefits and risks (top-down approach)
Step 6	*Calculation of the weighted scores at each level and calculation of the overall weighted scores*
	(1) normalization of the weights of the criteria at all levels (the total sum of all weights should equal 100, but the ratios between the weights should be preserved) (2) for each option, multiplication of the score of each criterion with its normalized weight; calculation of the overall preference score for each option which is the sum of the weighted scores
Step 7	*Conduction of a sensitivity analysis*
	Variation of the weight and/or the score on any criterion and assessment of its impact on the overall benefit–risk preference score

the next sections. At the end of each section the subject step is summarized as shown in Table 5.1.

Step 1: Establishment of the decision context

The decision context is relatively straightforward and has essentially been described earlier. Currently no validated and well-accepted models exist to conduct a benefit–risk assessment of medicines, either in the context of the approval of new medicines by the regulatory authorities, or in the context of the re-assessment of marketed medicines by regulatory authorities when a new safety issue surfaces. Therefore a new model was developed, based on a number of prerequisites identified earlier in this chapter. The overall goal of developing the new model is to enhance the process of trading off the benefits and risks of a given medicine, and thus to facilitate decisions about allowing or maintaining medicines on the market in case the benefit–risk balance is positive.

As indicated in Chapter 1, a separate benefit–risk assessment should be conducted for each indication, because medicines are clinically tested for each indication separately (Spilker, 1994; Beckmann, 1999). The efficacy and thus the benefits of a medicine in one indication are not the same as in another indication, and, similarly, the safety is not necessarily comparable, as the dosage might be different for different indications. This was further elaborated in Chapter 2 in which three prerequisites for benefit–risk assessment were identified, which define the scope of the assessment: the indication; the dosage for that particular indication; and the contraindications, as established in the product label. Thus, during the first step of the construction of the model these three specific pieces of information, established in the proposed labelling of the medicine, should be identified.

Step 1 *Establishment of the decision context*
Identification of the indication, the dosage for that indication, the contraindications, and the other critical safety wording in the proposed product label of the subject medicine.

Step 2: Identification of the options to be appraised

In contrast to most other problems for which MCDA is used as a decision tool, there is essentially only one option to be appraised – one medicine – for which the decision is either that the benefit–risk balance is positive (the benefits outweigh the risks), or negative (the risks outweigh the benefits). Also, there are no monetary objectives involved. However, for comparison purposes, the comparator(s) used in clinical trials serve as the other option(s). As will be discussed in the next section, the criteria used for judging the new medicine will therefore also be applied to the efficacy and safety data generated in the clinical trials for the active comparator(s) and/or for placebo (or exceptionally to the option of no treatment, for example for oncology medicines). This approach is consistent with the concept described in Chapter 1 that the availability of alternative therapies should be considered in benefit–risk assessment, and that the interpretation of the benefits and risks of medicines always involves a comparison.

   Step 2   *Identification of the options to be appraised*

       (1) the medicine being assessed
       (2) the comparators (active comparator and/or placebo) used in the pivotal clinical trials.

Step 3: Identification and organization of the criteria

Step 3.1: Identification of the criteria for assessing the consequences for each option

According to Belton and Stewart (2002), the following considerations are relevant in identifying the criteria for assessing the consequences of each option.

1. *Value relevance*: it must be ensured that each criterion is relevant for and linked to the higher level goals.

2. *Understandability*: it is important that there is a shared understanding of each criterion.

3. *Measurability*: MCDA implies some degree of measurement of the performance of each option against the specified criteria, and it must thus be possible to specify this in a consistent manner.

4. *Non-redundancy*: it must be addressed whether there is more than one criterion measuring the same factor. As a general rule, it is better to combine similar criteria in a single concept.

5. *Judgemental independence*: it must be assured that all criteria are mutually preference independent, i.e. the preference scores that are assigned on one criterion are unaffected by the preference scores on the other criteria. For example, although a correlation exists in the real world between the overall incidence of adverse effects and the incidence of serious adverse effects, a preference score can be given for the incidence of serious adverse effects without knowing the overall incidence of

adverse effects. Thus, preferences are mutually independent even though correlation exists in the real world.

6. *Balancing completeness and conciseness*: completeness, or exhaustiveness, and conciseness are potentially conflicting requirements. It is nevertheless important that all critical aspects of the problem are captured, but also that the model is concise, i.e. keeping the level of detail to the minimum required. A model that would be too comprehensive could be very complicated and time-consuming to use in practice, and therefore defeat the purpose of being a decision aid.

7. *Operationality*: associated with the need to achieve a balance between completeness and conciseness in terms of the criteria being selected, it is important that the model is usable with reasonable effort.

The identification of the criteria was done and described in Chapter 2 based on a review of the EU, US and ICH guidelines, complemented by a detailed review of the literature. Confirmation about the value of each criterion was sought by carrying out a pilot study involving senior people from the industry and senior people from regulatory authorities who were asked to confirm the usefulness of each criterion for a benefit–risk assessment. The identified criteria are the following.

- Benefit criteria:

   1. Efficacy versus comparator and its clinical relevance (for each pivotal trial)

   2. Design, conduct and statistical adequacy of the trial (for each pivotal trial)

   3. Clinical relevance of the primary endpoints (for each pivotal trial)

   4. Representativeness of the studied population for the population targeted in the label (for each pivotal trial)

   5. Statistical significance of the efficacy results (for each pivotal trial)

   6. Evidence for the efficacy in relevant subgroups (for each pivotal trial)

   7. Efficacy as given by the results of the non-primary endpoints (for each pivotal trial);

   8. Efficacy as given by the results of the relevant non-pivotal trials and extensions

9. Anticipated patient compliance in clinical practice

10. Clustering (consistency) of results of the pivotal trials.

- Risk criteria:

   1. Overall incidence of adverse effects

   2. Overall incidence of serious adverse effects

   3. Discontinuation rate due to adverse effects

   4. Incidence, seriousness, duration and reversibility of specific adverse effects

   5. Safety in subgroups

   6. Interactions with other drugs and food

   7. Potential for off-label use leading to safety hazards

   8. Potential for non-demonstrated additional risk due to limitations of clinical trials and/or length of patient exposure

   9. Potential for non-demonstrated additional risk due to safety issues observed in preclinical safety studies but not in humans

   10. Potential for non-demonstrated additional risk due to safety issues observed with other medicines of the same pharmacological class.

All these benefit and risk criteria comply in principle with the general considerations for identifying the relevant criteria as described above, with the exception of the five benefit criteria listed below which are not measurable because they do not allow for the options to be differentiated. They will however be taken into account during the weighting process (Step 5). These criteria can be considered as 'confidence criteria' as they relate primarily to the level of confidence that one has in the results of a pivotal trial, or in the consistency of the results of multiple trials, and they are as follows:

- design, conduct and statistical adequacy of the trial (for each pivotal trial)

- clinical relevance of the primary endpoints (for each pivotal trial)

- representativeness of the studied population for the population targeted in the label (for each pivotal trial)

- statistical significance of the efficacy results (for each pivotal trial)

- clustering (consistency) of results of the pivotal trials.

Step 3.2: Organization of the criteria in high-level and lower-level objectives in the hierarchy

There are different methodologies or schools of thought of MCDA for elaborating the different criteria in the model structure. The extent and the way in which the criteria are incorporated differ between these methodologies (Belton and Stewart, 2002). The easiest and most suitable way of organizing the benefit and risk criteria is constructing a value tree, which clusters the criteria in a hierarchical way. The objective of creating such a value tree should be a clear and simple representation of the problem and at the same time adequately capturing the issues.

A value tree for the benefit–risk balance of medicines was created (Figure 5.1), in which 'Benefits' and 'Risks' were established as the first-level criteria. With regard to benefit, since there is usually more than one pivotal clinical trial (at a minimum two and quite often more), a separate tree was created for each trial as a second-level criterion, which encompasses the three third-level criteria that are relevant to each pivotal trial. The two other benefit-criteria were clustered in a second-level criterion entitled 'Other benefit criteria'. The 10 risk criteria were clustered in three second-level criteria ('Adverse effects', 'Other risk criteria', and 'Potential for non-demonstrated additional risk'), which made the risk tree more manageable given the high number of risk criteria. Constructing the value tree in this way also provided assurance that it is symmetric and that the 'Benefits' arm and the 'Risks' arm both have two levels of sub-criteria, which facilitates the weighting process (Step 5).

Step 3   *Identification of the benefit and risk criteria and organization in a value tree*

(1)   identification of the pivotal clinical trials and their primary endpoints
(2)   drawing of the value tree as in Figure 5.1.

Step 4: Assessment of the expected performance of each option against the criteria

Step 4.1: Description of the consequences of the options

As described in Step 2, the consequences are straightforward and are that the benefit–risk balance of the medicine under examination is either positive (the benefits outweigh the risks), or negative (the risks outweigh the benefits). The more complicated issue is

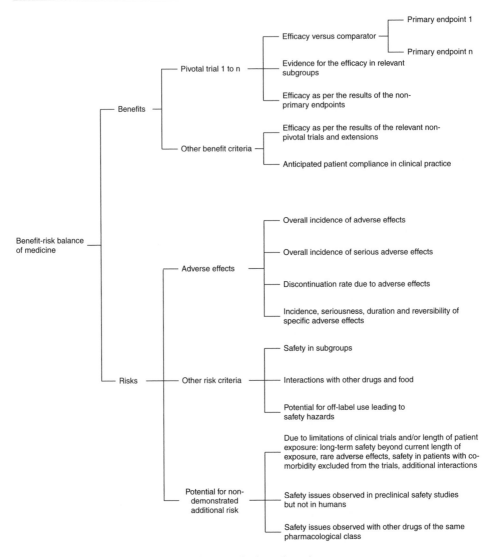

Figure 5.1   Value tree for benefit–risk assessment

to identify the dataset which will be used for scoring on each of the criteria for the medicine under examination and for the active comparator and/or placebo. Whilst for the benefit–risk assessment of new medicines the relevant data will be easy to identify and retrieve from the marketing authorization application, this may be more difficult for the post-marketing re-assessment of medicines, where there is usually no dossier that includes all safety and efficacy data. Thus, questions which will have to be addressed include the following:

- which are the pivotal trials?

- which are the relevant non-pivotal trials and extension studies?

- from which dataset can the overall incidence of adverse effects, the overall incidence of serious adverse effects, and the discontinuation rate due to adverse effects be retrieved?

Step 4.2: Scoring of the options on the criteria

Step 4.2 pertains to scoring the relevant available data on each of the criteria. Scoring is the process of assessing the performance of each of the options against the relevant criteria by assigning a numerical value (Belton and Stewart, 2002). If the criteria are structured as a value tree then the options must be scored against each of the bottom-level criteria of the tree. The performance of each of the options against the relevant criteria needs to be assessed on an interval scale of measurement, i.e. a scale on which the difference between points is the important factor. To construct a scale it is necessary to define two reference points and to allocate numerical values to these points. These are often taken to be the bottom and top of the scale, to which values of respectively 0 and 100 are assigned. However, other reference points and other values can be used. Two different scales should be distinguished.

- Fixed scales, of which the endpoints may be defined by the ideal and the worst conceivable performance on the particular criterion, or by the best and worst performance which could realistically occur. The definition of a fixed scale requires more work than a relative preference scale, which is described below. However, it has the advantages that it is more general than a relative preference scale and that it can be defined before the consideration of specific options. This latter consideration also means that it is possible to define weights for each of the criteria (Step 5) before the scoring of the options.

- Relative preference scales, which are scales anchored at their ends by the most and least preferred options on a criterion (which are assigned a score of 100 and 0, respectively). The preference score for each other option is then calculated in proportion to the least preferred and most preferred option. The use of relative preference scales permits a relatively quick assessment of values and can be very useful for an initial assessment of the problem.

With regard to fixed scales, once the reference points of the scale have been determined, consideration must be given to how other scores are to be assessed. This can be done in the following three ways (Belton and Stewart, 2002).

- *Definition of a partial value function*: an appropriate quantitative scale is identified which is closely related to the decision maker's values. This value function is usually linear, but can also be non-linear. For example, for a criterion such as distance from the railway station in choosing a house, a buyer might wish to be neither too close to the station (because of noise or other disruption), nor too far (to allow for convenient access). In such cases a non-linear value function, also called a piecewise value function, should be developed. Several methods exist for this purpose. If it is not possible to identify an appropriate quantitative scale, the construction of a qualitative value scale will be required.

- *Construction of a qualitative value scale*: often it is not possible to find a measurable attribute which captures a criterion. In such circumstances it is necessary to construct an appropriate qualitative scale. A number of methods exist to establish such scales and to subsequently convert and normalize the scale to a 0–100 quantitative scale.

- *Direct rating of the options*: this can be viewed as the construction of a value scale, but confined to defining only the endpoints of the scale. Thus, no attempt is made to define a scale which characterizes performance independently of the options being evaluated. A number is specified, or the position on a visual analogue scale is identified, which reflects the value of an option in relation to the specified reference points. Often the method of pairwise comparisons of the options is used to establish the options on the scale and to check consistency of the judgements.

For the purpose of constructing the model for benefit–risk assessment of medicines, fixed scales were used. A scale from 0 (usually defined as the minimal acceptable) to 100 (usually defined as the maximum technically feasible) was used to score each criterion. The 'least preferred' (score of 0) and 'most preferred' (score of 100) were defined for each criterion (Table 5.2) and represent the personal view of the author. Some of these definitions should be fine-tuned for each therapeutic class of products, as detailed in the footnote to the table, and the definitions below provide a general guidance in this respect. For the criteria for which numerical data are available, partial value functions can be defined and the scores can be linearly transformed into 0–100 value scales. For example, if the least preferred option for the criterion 'overall incidence of adverse effects' is 35%, and the most preferred option 5%, an incidence of 20% would receive a score of 50. The benefit and risk criteria for which such partial value functions can usually be defined are: efficacy in terms of primary endpoint, evidence for the efficacy in relevant subgroups, efficacy as per the results of non-primary endpoints, overall incidence of adverse effects, overall incidence of serious adverse effects, and discontinuation rate due to adverse effects. Direct rating of the options can be used for the other criteria, although ideally it should be attempted to develop partial value functions or, if not feasible, possibly qualitative value scales. For

Table 5.2 Least and most preferred scores for each benefit and risk criterion

	Least preferred	Most preferred
Benefit criteria		
Efficacy versus comparator in terms of primary endpoint (should be assessed separately for each primary endpoint of a given trial)	Efficacy equal to placebo in terms of the primary endpoint; Efficacy inferior to the active comparator in terms of the primary endpoint in a non-inferiority or equivalence trial, or similar to the comparator in a superiority trial	Efficacy in terms of the primary endpoint the best that can be expected for this kind of disease versus placebo[a] Efficacy in terms of the primary endpoint significantly superior to the active comparator which is considered the gold standard[a]
Evidence for the efficacy in relevant subgroups	Efficacy results as per the primary endpoint(s) in one or more specific subgroups equal to placebo; Efficacy in one or more subgroups inferior to the active comparator in a non-inferiority or equivalence trial, or similar to the comparator in a superiority trial	Efficacy results as given by the primary endpoint(s) are fully confirmed in each relevant subgroup
Efficacy as given by the results of the non-primary endpoints	One or more non-primary endpoints are considered to be clinically important but the results are equal to placebo, or inferior to the active comparator in a non-inferiority or equivalence trial, or inferior or similar to the comparator in a superiority trial	One or more non-primary endpoints are considered to be clinically important and the efficacy results of these non-primary endpoints are similar or exceed the results of the primary endpoints
Efficacy as per the results of the relevant non-pivotal trials and extensions	The results of the non-pivotal trials and extension trials are considered to be clinically important but are significantly worse than the results of the pivotal trials	The results of non-pivotal trials and extension trials are similar or superior to the results of the pivotal trials
Anticipated patient compliance in clinical practice	The pharmaceutical dosage form and/or the dosing frequency are inconvenient and will lead to a very significant number of patients being non-compliant, which will cause efficacy and/or safety issues	The pharmaceutical form and dosing frequency are optimal for the population and disease being treated

Table 5.2   (Continued)

	Least preferred	Most preferred
Risk criteria		
Overall incidence of adverse effects	Unacceptably high incidence of adverse effects[a]	Incidence of adverse effects is similar to placebo
Overall incidence of serious adverse effects	Unacceptably high incidence of serious adverse effects[a]	Incidence of serious adverse effects is similar to placebo
Discontinuation rate due to adverse effects	Unacceptably high incidence of discontinuation rate due to adverse effects[a]	Discontinuation rate due to adverse effects is similar to placebo
Incidence, seriousness, duration and reversibility of specific adverse effects	One or more adverse effects are unacceptably severe in terms of incidence, seriousness, duration and/or reversibility	No specific adverse effects of concern
Safety in population subgroups	The safety in one or more specific subgroups (e.g. female, black people) is clinically significantly worse than the safety in the general population studied, leading to an unacceptable risk in this or these subgroups	No particular safety issue identified in subgroup analyses and no theoretical reason to believe that there should be an issue
Interactions with other drugs and food	The drug has unmanageable interactions with other drugs or food leading to unacceptable safety issues	No clinically significant interactions with other drugs and food
Potential for off-label use leading to safety hazards	Very high likelihood for off-label use which will lead to unacceptable safety hazards due to (1) the use of the medicine outside the indication and/or dosage recommendation (possibly leading to an overdose), (2) the use of the medicine in situations where it is contraindicated (including pregnancy and lactation), (3) non-compliance with labelled precautions and warnings with regard to interactions, pregnancy and lactation, and driving and operating machines.	No theoretical grounds to believe that there will be significant off-label use, or off-label use would lead to no safety hazards
Due to limitations of clinical trials and/or length of patient exposure: long-term safety beyond current length of	Clinical trials and patient exposure data are insufficient to determine that there is an acceptable risk with regard to	Clinical trials and patient exposure data are sufficient to exclude any new safety hazards

exposure, rare adverse effects, safety in patients with comorbidity factors excluded from the trials, additional interactions	the unknowns for long-term safety, rare adverse effects, safety in patients with comorbidity and additional interactions	
Safety issues observed in preclinical safety studies but not in humans	Unacceptable safety issues observed in preclinical safety studies and theoretical basis to believe that these will also occur in humans	No safety issues observed in preclinical safety studies that could have relevance in humans
Safety issues observed with other drugs of the same pharmacological class	Unacceptable safety issues with other medicines of the same class and theoretical basis to believe that these issues could occur as well with the medicine under review	No particular safety issues observed with other medicines of the same class

[a] This must be specifically defined for each medicine under review according to the nature of the medicine and the disease for which it is indicated.

example, for the criterion 'potential for non-demonstrated additional risk due to limitations of clinical trials and/or length of patient exposure' it may be possible to develop, depending on the medicine under discussion, a partial value function based on patient-years of exposure. Whatever scales are used, they should be clinically relevant and consistent with the treatment expectations in the target population (Chuang-Stein *et al*, 2008).

As an alternative to fixed scales, relative preference scales can be used when there are at least three options to be assessed (e.g. the medicine under examination, the active comparator, and placebo). This is an easier way of scoring than by using fixed scales, because there is no need to define the scales, but as mentioned above the downside is that at least three options should be available for scoring, which is not always the case.

Step 4.3: Checking of the consistency of the scores on each criterion

Since the initial assessment of scores often reveals inconsistencies, both within and between criteria, consistency should be checked, which is usually accomplished during the process of assessing scores (Department for Transport, Local Government and the Regions, 2000). Several iterations of going over the scores assigned to the different options and of pairwise comparisons between the options may be needed until there is sufficient consistency. These pairwise comparisons are done by comparing the ratios of the differences in the scores between the options, for example the difference in the scores between options A and B is compared with the difference in the scores between options B and C.

Step 4   *Assessment of the performance of each option against the criteria*

(1) identification of the relevant data including the non-pivotal trials and extension studies, and the safety dataset
(2) construction of the scale for each criterion (partial value functions for selected criteria, direct rating for the other criteria), and scoring of each option on each criterion
(3) checking of the consistency of the scores on each criterion.

Step 5: Assignment of weights for each criterion to reflect their relative importance to the decision

In MCDA, weights are used to reflect the relative importance of criteria (Belton and Stewart, 2002). The weight assigned to a criterion is essentially a scaling factor which relates scores on that criterion to scores on all other criteria. Thus if criterion A has a weight which is twice that of criterion B, this should be interpreted that 10 value points on criterion A is valued the same as 20 value points on criterion B. This concept is referred to as 'swing weighting', which is thus a method of eliciting relative weights on different criteria. Swing weighting requires judgements of the swing in preference from 0 to 100 on one preference scale as compared to the 0–100 swing on another preference scale. The judgements are made by considering the difference between 0 and 100 positions, and how much that difference matters. Those two considerations take account of the range of real-world difference on the criteria (i.e. the scale being used), and the importance of that difference to achieving the overall objective (i.e. the intrinsic importance of the criterion). If an intrinsically important criterion does not differentiate much between the options, i.e. if the minimum and maximum points on the value scale correspond to similar levels of performance, then that criterion may be ranked quite low. For example, cost is considered to be important in purchasing a car. However, when a shortlist of five cars is made that only differ in price by €500, cost becomes an unimportant criterion in making the final choice, and may be given a minimal weight.

Thus, swing-weighting results in ratio-scale numbers that reflect the relative importance of the criteria. In practical terms, the criterion with the biggest swing in preference from 0 to 100 (the largest difference that matters) is identified first. This criterion is given a weight of 100 and becomes the standard. All other criteria are compared to this standard. For example, the criterion that is judged to be next in relative importance can be given a weight of 90.

When the problem is structured as a multi-level value tree, as is the case here, it is useful to define relative weights and cumulative weights (Belton and Stewart, 2002).

Relative weights are assessed within families of criteria, i.e. criteria sharing the same parent. Within each family, the weights assigned to each criterion as per the method described in the previous paragraph are normalized to sum to 100. The cumulative weight of a criterion is the product of its relative weight and the relative weight of its parent, parent's parent, and so on to the top of the three. By definition, the cumulative weights of all bottom-level criteria sum to 100. The cumulative weight of a parent criterion is the total of the cumulative weights of its descendants. If the value tree does not have too many leaves, then weights can be assessed by directly comparing all bottom-level criteria (Belton and Stewart, 2002). Weights at higher levels of the tree are then determined by adding the weights of all members of a family to give the cumulative weight of the parent. Normalized weights are determined by normalizing the weights of family members to sum to 100. For larger models it is easier to begin by assessing relative weights within families of criteria. Weights at higher levels of the value tree can be assessed top-down or bottom-up. The top-down approach assesses relative weights by working from the top of the tree downwards. However, the difficulty with this approach is that in comparing two higher level criteria a swing from 0 to 100 should be considered on all sub-criteria of the two higher level criteria. The bottom-up approach begins by assessing relative weights within families which contain only bottom-level criteria and then carrying out cross family comparisons, most often using one criterion from each family (usually the most highly weighted criterion in each family). This process will eventually give the cumulative weights of the bottom-level criteria which can be aggregated to higher levels as described above.

With regard to the benefit criteria, swing-weighting is conducted using a bottom-up approach as follows.

- The relative weights of the three second-level trial-specific benefit criteria are assigned using swing-weighting. If there would be more than one primary endpoint in a given trial (i.e. *n* primary endpoints), there will be a separate criterion pertaining to the efficacy results for each of the *n* primary endpoints, and each of the *n* criteria will be weighted separately. One of these *n* criteria will probably be the criterion with the biggest swing in preference and will be given a weight of 100. The two second-level criteria under the node 'Other benefit criteria' will be weighted separately, and one of these two criteria will be given a weight of 100 against which the other criterion is compared.

- Next, the first-level benefit criteria are weighted, which includes weighting the relative importance of each trial as well as the node 'other benefit criteria'. First, the criterion with the biggest swing in preference is identified, which is probably one of the pivotal trials. Specific criteria can be established to decide on the relative importance of trials, for example the number of patients included in the trial, the duration of the trial and/or the inclusion of both a placebo and an active comparator arm (if for example the other pivotal trials do not include placebo and an active comparator). In addition, the criteria previously identified as providing confidence in the results of a trial should also be taken into account:

► Design, conduct and statistical adequacy of the trial;

► Clinical relevance of the primary endpoints;

► Representativeness of the studied population for the population targeted in the label;

► Statistical significance of the efficacy results;

► Clustering (consistency) of results of the pivotal trials.

However, the factors to be taken into account to decide on the relative importance of the pivotal trials should not pertain to the actual outcomes of the trials since these trial results are already incorporated in the model during the scoring of the trial-specific criteria. Next, the weights of the other first-level benefit criteria are determined using the bottom-up approach.

With regard to the risk criteria, weights can be assessed by directly comparing all bottom-level risk criteria. It is in principle not required to weight separately the first-level criteria and the second-level criteria using a bottom-up or top-down approach. The single criterion for which the difference between least preferred and most preferred matters most, is most likely the incidence/seriousness/duration/reversibility of specific adverse effects, which again is given a weight of 100, to which all other risk criteria are compared for assigning them a weight. Weights at higher levels of the tree (i.e. 'Adverse effects', 'Other risk criteria', and 'Potential for non-demonstrated additional risk') are then determined by adding the weights of all members of a family to give the cumulative weight of the parent.

As a final step, it is required to judge the relative difference between benefits and risks in terms of weight, by using the top-down approach. For example, benefit overall can be assigned a weight of 60, and risk overall a weight of 40. This allows taking into account the relative importance of benefits versus risks, which is different from one therapeutic area to another (Miller, 1993; Meyboom and Egberts, 1999; Arlett, 2001). For example, for anticancer products the emphasis in the assessment lies on the benefits much more than on the risks because cancer is a life-threatening disease for which the risk due to the medicine is not very important given the high risk of dying from the disease. At the other end of the spectrum, for OTC medicines risk is very important since, for the kind of minor illnesses for which OTC medicines are used, only minimal side effects are acceptable to physicians and patients. Thus, in fact this process allows taking into account what some authors have called the third dimension with regard to benefit–risk assessment, that is, the seriousness of the disease (benefit and risk of the medicine being the other two dimensions), which influences the generally acceptable magnitude of benefits and risks of a medicine. However, this procedure tends to bias the weights if there are many more criteria under one of the branches than under the other. Therefore, an alternative approach for assigning the relative weights of benefits and risks is comparing the one benefit criterion assigned the highest weight with the one risk criterion assigned the highest weight, by considering the difference between 0 and 100 positions for both criteria, and how much that difference matters.

Step 5   *Assignment of a weight to each criterion using swing-weighting*

    (1) assignment of the relative weights to the bottom-level benefit criteria under each pivotal trial and under the 'other benefit criteria'

    (2) assignment of the relative weights of the pivotal trials and the 'other benefit criteria', taking into account the trial confidence criteria (bottom-up approach)

    (3) assignment of the relative weights to the risk criteria

    (4) assignment of the relative weights to the benefits and risks (top-down approach).

Step 6: Calculation of the weighted scores at each level in the hierarchy and calculation of the overall weighted scores

The weights of all first-level, second-level and third-level criteria are normalized, so that the total sum of all weights equals 100, but preserves the ratios between the different weights at all levels (Department for Transport, Local Government and the Regions, 2000). Then, for each option the score of each criterion is multiplied by its normalized weight. The overall preference score for each option is simply the weighted average of its scores on all the criteria.

The sum of the weighted scores is calculated for benefits, for risks, and for benefits plus risks. The final benefit–risk score for each option can also be expressed as a ratio by dividing the weighted score for benefits by the weighted score for risks. These results will show whether the benefits, risks, and benefits plus risks of the medicine under assessment outweigh the benefits, risks, and benefits plus risks of the other options, which are usually placebo and/or an active comparator, and by how much.

In summary, letting the preference score for option I on criterion j be represented by s_{ij} and the weight for each criterion by w_j, then for n criteria the overall score for each option S_i is given by the following algorithm:

$$S_i = w_1 s_{i1} + w_2 s_{i2} + w_n s_{in} = \sum_{j=1}^{n} w_i s_{ij} \quad \text{with} \quad \sum_{j=1}^{n} w = 100$$

Step 6   *Calculation of the weighted scores at each level and calculation of the overall weighted scores*

(1) normalization of the weights of the criteria at all levels (the total sum of all weights should equal 100, but the ratios between the weights should be preserved)

(2) for each option, multiplication of the score of each criterion with its normalized weight; calculation of the overall preference score for each option which is the sum of the weighted scores.

Step 7: Examination of the result and conduction of sensitivity analysis

A sensitivity analysis should be carried out to investigate whether the conclusions reached in Step 6 are robust or if they are sensitive to changes in aspects of the model (Belton and Stewart, 2002). Changes may be made to investigate the significance of missing information, to explore the effect of uncertainties about values and priorities, or to offer a different perspective on the problem. In practical terms, a sensitivity analysis should be performed in order to optimize the weights. A sensitivity analysis enables the weight on any criterion to be varied throughout its entire range from 0 to 100, and to assess its impact on the overall benefit–risk preference score for each option. It is also possible to vary the scores during a sensitivity analysis. This may in particular be relevant when qualitative value scales, direct rating of the options, or relative preference scales are used, because these scoring methods require a judgement in contrast to partial value functions.

A sensitivity analysis can also be applied to make the final decision on the population in which the right benefit–risk balance is achieved, and to establish it in the label. For this purpose one or more of the three parameters which define the scope of the assessment can either be broadened or further restricted, i.e. the indication, the dosage for that particular indication, or the contraindications. For example, if the label would be broadened to a wider population in terms of a less restricted indications wording or less contraindications, the scores and possibly the weights on some of the benefit and risk criteria would vary, which would have an impact on the overall preference score.

Step 7   *Conduction of a sensitivity analysis*:
Variation of the weight and/or the score on any criterion and assessment of its impact on the overall benefit–risk preference score

5.6 APPLICABILITY OF THE NEW MODEL

Introduction

An existing medicine (i.e. MAXALT [rizatriptan], a 5-HT$_{1B/1D}$ agonist for the treatment of migraine) was used to illustrate the applicability of the new model developed in the previous section. This medicine was also used as an example in Chapter 3 with regard to the applicability of the existing models for benefit–risk assessment. The MCDA software Hiview 3 described in Chapter 4 was used to calculate the overall preference score for each option and to conduct a sensitivity analysis. The scores and weights assigned in this example represent the opinion of the author and were not validated by other experts. Nevertheless, this example provided valuable experience on the applicability of the model.

Example: Rizatriptan

The decision context (Step 1) for using the MCDA-based model on this medicine was to illustrate that rizatriptan (in a dose of 10 mg) has a positive benefit–risk balance compared to the other options that will be appraised, based on the data available in the original marketing authorization application. The indication for MAXALT in the EU is 'acute treatment of the headache phase of migraine attacks with or without aura'. The recommended dosage is 10 mg for adults 18 years of age and older (Electronic Medicines Compendium, 2004). Doses should be separated by at least 2 h; no more than two doses should be taken in any 24-h period. There were three pivotal phase III studies that demonstrate the efficacy of rizatriptan 10 mg for the abortive treatment of migraine attacks in a large number of outpatients (Medicines Evaluation Board, 1999). Pivotal trial #1 was a double-blind random study which examined the efficacy of rizatriptan 5 mg and 10 mg for the acute treatment of migraine and migraine recurrence in a total of 1218 treated patients. The study included initial doses of rizatriptan 5 mg ($n = 458$), rizatriptan 10 mg ($n = 456$), and placebo ($n = 304$), followed by treatment with up to two additional doses for recurrence within 24 h. The primary efficacy comparisons were the percentages of patients reporting pain relief at 2 h following rizatriptan 5 mg (62%) and 10 mg (71%) versus placebo (35%). Pivotal trial #2 was a double-blind randomised study which examined the efficacy of rizatriptan 10 mg versus placebo for the acute treatment of up to four consecutive migraine attacks in a total of 407 treated patients. The primary efficacy comparison was the percent of patients reporting pain relief at 2 h following rizatriptan 10 mg (77%) versus placebo (37%) during the first attack. Pivotal trial #3 was a double-blind randomised study which compared the efficacy of rizatriptan 5 mg and 10 mg to sumatriptan 100 mg for the acute treatment of migraine in a total of 1099 treated patients. The study included single doses of rizatriptan 5 mg ($n = 164$), rizatriptan 10 mg ($n = 387$), sumatriptan 100 mg ($n = 388$), and placebo ($n = 160$). The primary efficacy comparisons were: (1) the percentages of patients reporting pain relief at 2 h following rizatriptan 5 mg (60%) and 10 mg (67%) versus placebo (40%); and (2) time to relief within 2 h for rizatriptan 10 mg versus sumatriptan 100 mg (hazard ratio 1.17; 95% confidence interval = 0.98, 1.39). Thus, the other options to which rizatriptan will be compared are placebo and sumatriptan, since these were the comparator agents used in the above mentioned pivotal clinical trials (Step 2). Next, a value tree was established in Hiview 3 (Figure 5.2) based on the general value tree developed in the previous section. With regard to the benefit criteria, the three

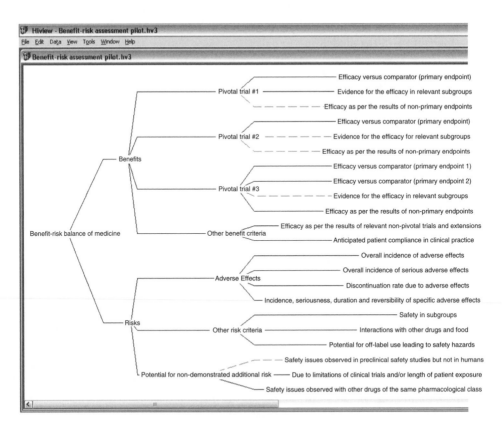

Figure 5.2   Value tree generated with Hiview 3 for rizatriptan

'pivotal trial' arms were included under the high-level criterion 'benefits', in addition to the 'other benefits criteria' arm (Step 3).

In Step 4, the scales for each of the criteria were established and the different options were scored accordingly. In this example, fixed scales were used because it would be difficult to use relative preference scales with only three options to be appraised. Partial value functions were defined for the following criteria.

- Efficacy versus comparator (in terms of the primary endpoint): the percentage of patients reporting pain relief at 2 h was used as the scale, with the percentage on placebo and 100% as respectively the least preferred and most preferred scores. This was the primary endpoint for all three pivotal trials, but for pivotal trial #3, a second primary endpoint was time to relief within 2 h. For this variable, the cumulative percentage of patients with first report of pain relief within 2 h was used as the scale, again with the percent on placebo and 100% as respectively the least preferred and most preferred scores.

- Overall incidence of adverse effects, overall incidence of serious adverse effects, and discontinuation rate due to adverse effects: the percentage of patients constituted the scale for these three criteria. The most preferred score for all three criteria was the incidence/discontinuation rate with placebo. In theory an incidence/discontinuation rate of 100% could be chosen as the least preferred score, but such a score is exaggerated from a practical clinical perspective and would construct a scale which would hardly discriminate between the different options. Since, based on the pooled safety database of all phase III trials, the percentages for all three options for these three criteria were between 0% and 11%, a more clinically meaningful scale is 0–20% for overall incidence of adverse effects, and 0–5% for overall incidence of serious adverse effects and for discontinuation rate due to adverse effects.

For all the other benefit and risk criteria the technique of direct rating of the options was applied. The least and most preferred options defined in Table 5.2 were used as a reference for the bottom and the top of the scales. For each criterion, the scale, its format and a short definition were entered in the Hiview 3 software. An example is provided in Figure 5.3. Next, the scores are entered for all three options on each criterion (Figure 5.4). Hiview 3 requires that each option is scored on each criterion. However, sumatriptan is not used as comparator agent in the pivotal trials #1 and #2, and scores can thus in principle not be attributed to the benefit criteria under these trial nodes. Using a conservative approach, sumatriptan was given the same score as rizatriptan on these criteria.

For pivotal trial pivotal trial #1, a score of 55 was assigned for rizatriptan on the criterion 'evidence for the efficacy in relevant subgroups', versus 100 for placebo.

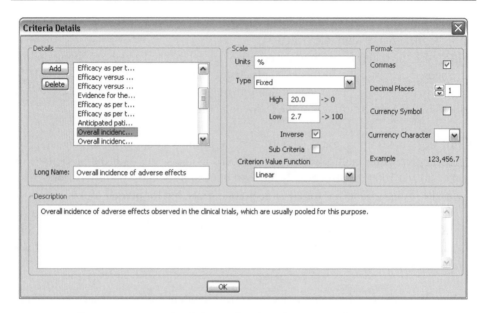

Figure 5.3   Example of criteria details with Hiview 3 for rizatriptan

Although there was no main effect of age, race, headache severity, presence/absence of aura, and use of concomitant medications in this trial, a score of 55 was justified because of a gender-by-treatment interaction. This interaction indicated that, in terms of pain relief at 2 h, the difference between rizatriptan and placebo was 58.8 % in males, whereas the difference was 32.1% in females (i.e. approx. 55% of the effect in males). This can be considered as a clinically significant issue given that migraine is more prevalent in females than in males. There were no clinically significant issues with regard to the efficacy in any subgroups in pivotal trials #2 and #3, and both rizatriptan and sumatriptan were thus given a score of 100, versus 0 for placebo, on these criteria. The results on the non-primary endpoints of pivotal trial #1 (i.e. pain-free at 2 h, use of escape medication, recurrence within 24 h, presence of associated symptoms, functional disability rating, satisfaction with medication, and 24 h quality of life) generally confirmed the results on the primary endpoint. Therefore a score of 100 was assigned to rizatriptan on this criterion, versus 0 to placebo. The same reasoning and scoring applied to pivotal trial #2. As a clinically significant difference was identified between rizatriptan and sumatriptan in pivotal trial #3 in terms of the key secondary endpoint pain free at 2 h, the results on this specific endpoint were used to create a partial value function. The pivotal trials #1 and #2 had an extension phase of up to 12 months duration, which showed that the likelihood of response within patients did not change over time – there was no evidence of tachyphylaxis. Hence, both rizatriptan and sumatriptan were given a

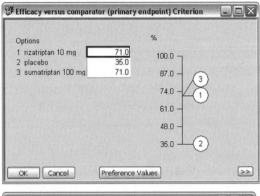

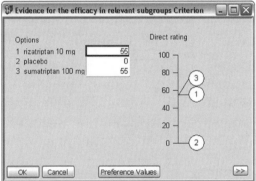

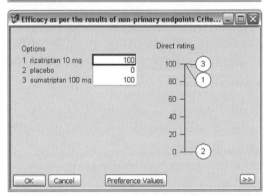

Figure 5.4
Scoring
of the options
on each criterion
with Hiview 3
for rizatriptan

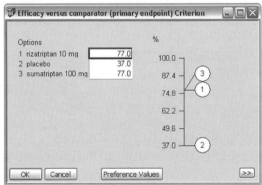

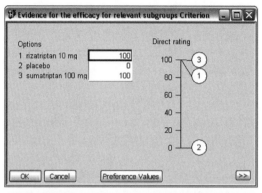

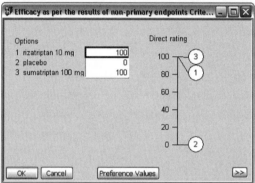

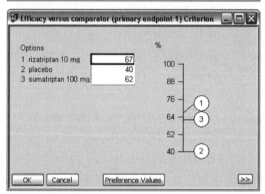

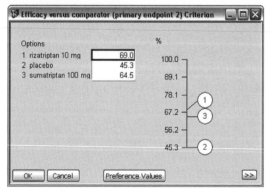

Figure 5.4
(Continued)

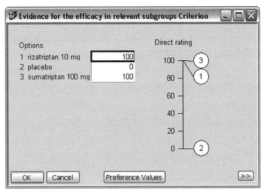

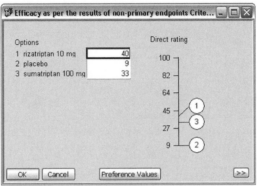

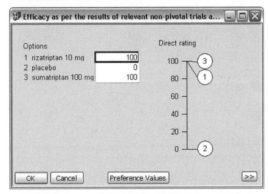

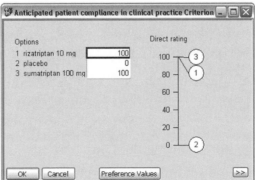

Figure 5.4
(Continued)

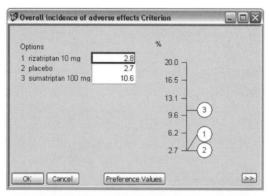

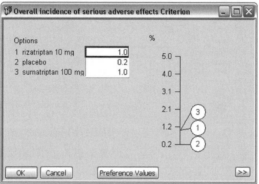

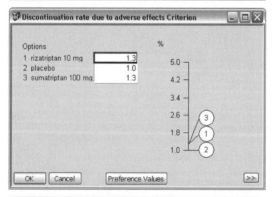

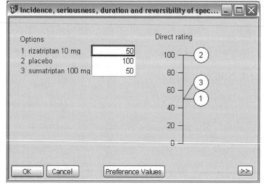

Figure 5.4
(Continued)

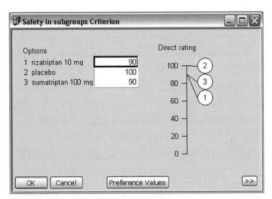

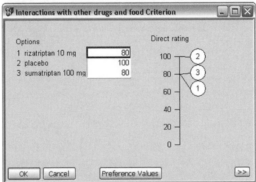

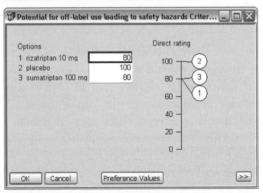

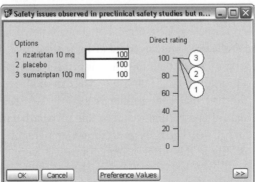

Figure 5.4
(Continued)

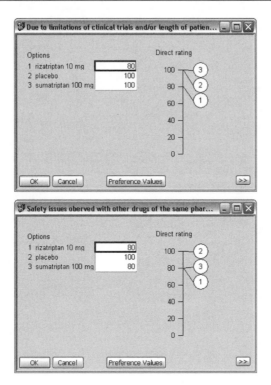

Figure 5.4
(Continued)

score of 100, and placebo a score of 0, on the criterion 'efficacy as per the results of relevant non-pivotal trials and extensions'. Both rizatriptan and sumatriptan were formulated as regular tablets to be administered in case of a migraine attack, and thus the same scores were given as on the previous criterion.

The most common drug-related adverse experiences in patients on rizatriptan 10 mg were dizziness (8%, versus 7% on sumatriptan 100 mg and 3% on placebo), somnolence (8%, versus 6% on sumatriptan 100 mg and 3% on placebo), and asthenia/ fatigue (5%, versus 6% on sumatriptan 100 mg and 1% on placebo). The percentage of patients on sumatriptan 100 mg with a drug-related event of chest pain was about the double of that for rizatriptan 10 mg (5% versus 3%, versus 1% on placebo). There were no specific drug-related serious adverse effects of concern noted in the safety database. However, myocardial ischaemia and myocardial infarction have been reported rarely with sumatriptan. Taking all these data together, it can for example be considered that rizatriptan has a safety profile which is half as good as that of placebo and should thus be assigned a score of 50, and that sumatriptan is slightly worse than rizatriptan only because of the rare events of myocardial ischemia and myocardial infarction, and should therefore receive a score of 40. There were no drug–demographic and disease interactions, and the safety profile in the different subgroups was very similar to the general safety profile. These same scores were therefore assigned as for the previous criterion. With regard to the criterion 'interactions with other drugs and food', there was one clinically significant interaction for rizatriptan 10 mg and one for sumatriptan 100 mg. The concomitant use of rizatriptan 10 mg and propranolol, which is used for migraine prophylaxis, lead to higher plasma concentrations of rizatriptan and there a dose of 5 mg should be used. The administration of ergotamine, which is also used to treat a migraine attack, should be separated from the intake of sumatriptan because of potential additive prolonged vasospastic reactions. Since both interactions are rather easy to manage, it was considered that both rizatriptan and sumatriptan should receive a score which was 4/5 of the score for placebo (i.e. 80). All triptans have a number of cardiovascular contra-indications because myocardial ischaemia and myocardial infarction occur rarely with sumatriptan and potentially also with other triptans. Because there was a doubt whether prescribers would fully comply with these contraindications and warnings, both riza-triptan and sumatriptan were given a score of 80, which is 4/5 of the score for placebo. There were no additional safety issues observed in preclinical safety studies that could be relevant to humans, and all three options were thus given a score of 100 on this criterion. Because rizatriptan was assessed based on the original dataset, which did not include post-marketing safety data, the patient exposure is much less than for sumatriptan and is therefore assigned a score of 75 versus 100 for sumatriptan and placebo. Finally, with regard to safety issues observed with other drugs of the same class, the concern of rare events of myocardial ischemia and myocardial infarction is real and may materialize during the commercialization of the medicine. A score of 75 versus 100 for sumatriptan and placebo can therefore be considered as justified.

Swing-weighting was applied for the weighting process in Step 5. First, the criteria for each of the three pivotal trials are weighted separately. For all three trials, the largest difference between the options that matters was 'efficacy versus the comparator (primary endpoint)', and was given a weight of 100 (Figure 5.5).

Pivotal trial #1	Weight	placebo rizatriptan 10 mg	triptan 100 mg	Cumulative Weight
Efficacy versus comparator (primary endpoint)*	100	55	0 55	9.0
Evidence for the efficacy in relevant subgroups*	50	55	0 55	4.5
Efficacy as per the results of non-primary endpoints*	0	100	0 100	0.0
TOTAL	150	55	0 55	13.5

Figure 5.5 Swing-weighting of the criteria under pivotal trial pivotal trial #1 with Hiview 3 for rizatriptan

In pivotal trial #1, the criterion 'evidence for the efficacy in relevant subgroups' was considered half as important as the first criterion, and the difference between the options mattered only half as much as for the first criterion. In pivotal trial #3, the 'efficacy of the results as per the non-primary endpoints' and the difference between the options on this criterion was considered to matter 4/5 as much as for the first criterion. All other criteria received a weight of 0 because they did not discriminate between rizatriptan and sumatriptan, and because the difference between rizatriptan and placebo did not really matter from a clinical perspective. With regard to the other benefit criteria, the 'efficacy as shown by the results of the relevant non-pivotal trials and extensions' was considered to be most important and given a weight of 100, whilst the 'anticipated patient compliance during market use' was considered to be unimportant because it did not discriminate between rizatriptan and placebo. Next, the four nodes under benefits were weighted. Based on the following factors pivotal trial #3 was assigned a weight of 100, in particular due to the fact that this trial included both a placebo and a sumatriptan arm, which was the contrasting factor with the other two trials:

- number of patients included in the trial, the duration of the trial, and the inclusion of both a placebo and an active comparator arm

- design, conduct and statistical adequacy of the trial

- clinical relevance of the primary endpoints

- representativeness of the studied population for the population targeted in the label

- statistical significance of the efficacy results

- clustering (consistency) of results of the pivotal trials.

The other two trials were assigned a weight of 70, and this judgement was facilitated by comparing the criterion with the highest swing for each trial and by assessing how much the difference between the options mattered versus the other criteria. The 'other benefit criteria' were assigned a weight of 20.

With regard to risks, the largest difference between the options that mattered (in particular between rizatriptan and placebo) was the 'incidence, seriousness, duration and reversibility of specific adverse effects'. The 'overall incidence of adverse effects' and the 'overall incidence of serious adverse effects' mattered slightly less but the difference between the options was nevertheless clinically significant, and therefore both criteria were given a weight of 80. All other risk criteria were considered to be less than half as important compared to the first criterion. Finally, for a disease such as migraine which is temporarily disabling for patients but not life-threatening, it can be considered that benefits are equally important to risks and that both should therefore receive the same weight overall.

In Step 6, Hiview 3 automatically calculates the normalized weights, which are expressed as cumulative weights (Figure 5.6). It then calculates the weighted scores, and eventually the sum of the weighted scores, which is also called the overall preference score, for each option. In this example, rizatriptan 10 mg was assigned an overall preference score of 67 (27.8 on benefits and 39.0 on risks), sumatriptan 100 mg a score of 61 (26.2 on benefits and 35.0 on risks), and placebo a score of 50 (0 on benefits and 50 on risks) (Figure 5.7). Thus, rizatriptan was slightly better than sumatriptan both in terms benefits and in terms of risks, and both were better than placebo in terms of benefits

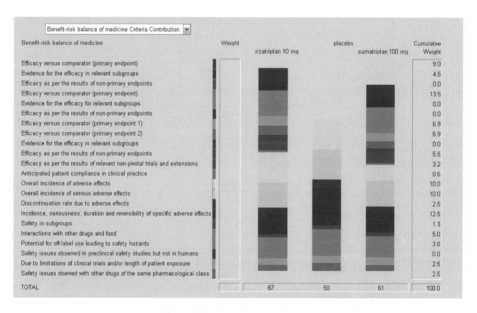

Figure 5.6   Normalised weights of all criteria with Hiview 3 for rizatriptan
Note: The normalised weights are listed in the right column.

In the final step (Step 7), a sensitivity analysis was conducted. For example, the overall weight on benefits would have to decrease to less than 30 for placebo to become the overall preferred option instead of rizatriptan (Figure 5.8). Similarly, the overall weight on risks would have to increase to more than 70 for placebo to become the preferred option instead of rizatriptan (Figure 5.9). It is also possible to

Benefit-risk balance of medicine	Weight rizatriptan 10 mg		placebo sumatriptan 100 mg		Cumulative Weight
Benefits	680	27.8	0.0	26.2	50.0
Risks	680	39.0	50.0	35.0	50.0
TOTAL	1360	67	50	61	100.0

Root Node Node Data

Benefit-risk balance of medicine Weighted Scores

Figure 5.7   Overall preference scores with Hiview 3 for rizatriptan

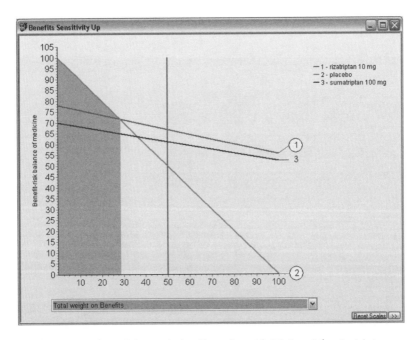

Figure 5.8   Sensitivity analysis of benefits with Hiview 3 for rizatriptan

assess the sensitivity of a specific criterion such as for example the 'incidence, seriousness, duration and reversibility of specific adverse effects'. The current cumulative weight of this criterion of 12.5 would have to increase to 35 for placebo to become the preferred option instead of rizatriptan (Figure 5.10). Decreasing the score of rizatriptan on this criterion from 50 to 20 would decrease the overall preference score of rizatriptan to 63, which is still slightly better than the overall score for sumatriptan

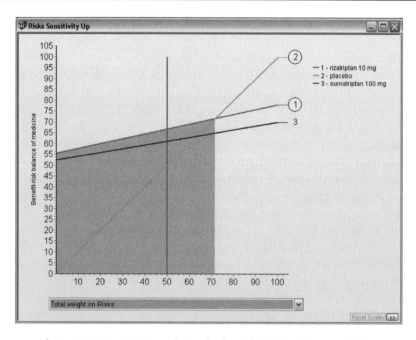

Figure 5.9 Sensitivity analysis of risks with Hiview 3 for rizatriptan

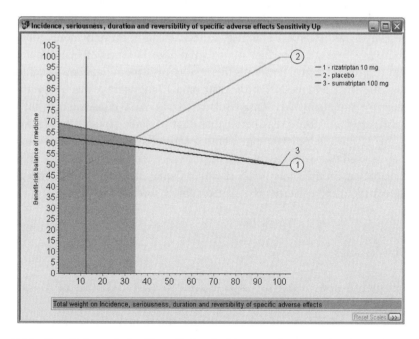

Figure 5.10 Sensitivity analysis of the criterion 'incidence, seriousness, duration and reversibility of specific adverse effects' with Hiview 3 for rizatriptan

Discussion

The above medicine served as an example to illustrate how the MCDA-based model is applied in practice using the Hiview 3 software. It was demonstrated that it is possible to enter real efficacy and safety data into the model, and eventually to obtain an overall benefit–risk score which distinguishes rizatriptan 10 mg from the other options (i.e. placebo and sumatriptan 100 mg). One assumption that had to be made was that the active comparator sumatriptan had the same score as rizatriptan on the criteria pertaining to the clinical trials in which sumatriptan was not included. A potential improvement with regard to the scoring would be to develop partial value functions for more criteria, instead of using direct scoring. The process of swing-weighting did not cause any specific problems. A weight of 0 was assigned to some criteria because they did not really matter within the scope of the example. Obviously that may not be the case for other medicines. Finally, it should be emphasized that all scores that were assigned by direct rating as well as all weights, represent the judgement of the author only, and would thus inevitably be different if other people would be involved in this exercise.

Specifically with regard to rizatriptan, a number of preliminary conclusions can be drawn, although a repetition of this test by other experts would be required to confirm these conclusions. As expected, both rizatriptan and sumatriptan were better than placebo in terms of benefits, and worse in terms of risks. This result is consistent with the fact that both medicines are licensed as first-line treatment for migraine (Physician's Desk Reference, 2008). In addition and more importantly, rizatriptan was slightly better than sumatriptan both in terms of benefits and risks. The latter results are consistent with the results of a meta-analysis which demonstrated that the NNT and the NNH for rizatriptan 10 mg were respectively lower and higher than for sumatriptan 100 mg (Belsey, 2001). As a consequence, the overall profile of rizatriptan 10 mg was better than that of sumatriptan 100 mg on a two-dimensional visual analogue graph. Thus, the results of this test suggest that the model can be used to assess the relative benefit–risk profile of a medicine compared to other medicines in the same pharmacological class, thereby providing a measure for the overall relative effectiveness of the subject medicine.

5.7   SUMMARY

In this chapter, a new model for assessing the benefit–risk balance of medicines based on MCDA was developed. It was demonstrated in detail through a seven-step approach how MCDA is used to construct the model. These seven steps were the following.

- Step 1: establish the decision context.

- Step 2: identify the options to be appraised (i.e. the medicine under discussion and usually either placebo and/or an active comparator).

- Step 3: identify the criteria (i.e. 5 benefit criteria and 10 risk criteria) and organize these criteria in a value tree.

- Step 4: establish fixed scales for all criteria and score the options on the criteria.

- Step 5: assign weights for each criterion by applying swing-weighting and using a bottom-up approach for the benefit criteria, direct weighting for the risk criteria, and a top-down approach for the benefits and risks overall.

- Step 6: normalize the weights, calculate the weighted scores at each level in the value tree and calculate the overall preference score for each option.

- Step 7: examine the results and conduct a sensitivity analysis by varying the weight on any criterion.

The model was applied to an existing medicine and it was demonstrated that it is possible to enter real efficacy and safety data into the model, and eventually to obtain a meaningful overall benefit–risk score.

In principle, this model complies with, or should be able to comply with the seven prerequisites which had been established for the new model. However, this will be further examined during the validation of the new model described below.

5.8   REVIEW OF THE MCDA MODEL

The above MCDA model was recently published (Mussen *et al.*, 2007) and was extensively reviewed and commented upon by a number of different stakeholders (Appendix 4). In addition, it was reviewed in the recent CHMP reflection paper on benefit–risk assessment methods (Appendix 3). In general, it is recognized that placing benefits and risks on a common scale and conducting a quantitative decision analysis remains difficult (Temple, 2007).

CHAPTER 6

A Future Framework for Benefit–Risk Appraisal of Medicines

6.1 BACKGROUND

In June 2008, the CMR International Institute for Regulatory Science held a workshop in Washington entitled 'Measuring Benefit and Balancing Risk: Strategies for the Benefit–risk Assessment of New Medicines in a Risk-Averse Environment'. This workshop brought together senior regulators from a number of authorities, executives from the pharmaceutical industry and academia to review the current studies, knowledge and experience in the development of a benefit–risk framework for the assessment of medicines. This chapter is based on the findings and the outcome of that workshop. A few months later, the Medicines and Healthcare products Regulatory Agency (MHRA) organized a forum with key stakeholders on the same theme, and came to similar conclusions (Appendix 6).

6.2 DEVELOPMENT OF A BENEFIT–RISK FRAMEWORK FOR REGULATORY REVIEW OF NEW MEDICINES

At this workshop, Theresa Mullin described how the FDA had established a new function entitled 'Planning and Business Informatics' concerned with long-term planning, modernization of the way FDA functions. A more systematic approach to the way FDA addresses benefit–risk assessment is part of this. Assessment with review staff in both CBER and CDER had provided an opportunity to examine the state of the art tools currently available and their applicability to the agency's work.

Benefit-Risk Appraisal of Medicines   Filip Mussen, Sam Salek, Stuart Walker
© 2009 John Wiley & Sons, Ltd

A single formalized way of expressing the benefit–risk balance could lose much of the valuable information that is currently provided for clinicians and patients in the labelling and that better measures are needed for measuring 'benefit' as opposed to 'efficacy' and that improved, standardised tools are needed for the evaluation of economic and quality of life benefits (CMR International Institute Workshop, Theresa Mullin 2008).

At this meeting Victor Raczkowski from Solvay outlined the need for a more formal approach to benefit–risk frameworks. Agreed frameworks will enhance the quality, effectiveness, and efficiency by which patients have access to high-quality therapies with favourable benefit–risk profiles and that affect patients' lives in meaningful and positive ways.

Not only has the environment for research and development of new medicines changed but the perception of risks has also changed. The thresholds for approval and market access are perceived as becoming higher and more difficult to overcome and there is a renewed and heightened focus on safety, with less willingness to accept uncertainty.

Increased requirements and the challenging practicalities of product development have led to the well-documented increasing timelines and escalating costs, with fewer new chemical entities being approved for marketing. Meanwhile, despite greater transparency and publication of data in the public domain (e.g. www.clinicaltrials.gov) the public perception of the pharmaceutical industry and its regulators remains negative. Product withdrawals are met with a public outcry, questions of assigning blame and suspicions that data has been concealed.

The adoption of benefit–risk frameworks should stimulate a 'cascade' of improvements in the development and review process leading to better informed, higher quality, and more consistent benefit–risk decision-making underpinned by:

- data: improved knowledge of the underlying science and increased availability of high-quality data upon which well-informed benefit–risk decisions are based

- analysis and interpretation: increased use of suitable metrics and greater consistency in the analyses from which valid benefit–risk inferences can be made

- communication on how decisions are made: greater alignment, confidence and understanding among all stakeholders.

Increased clarity and transparency in the process of decision making is essential to the acceptance of the underlying assumptions, values, perceptions, and judgements that are used in benefit–risk assessments. In establishing good practices and a benefit–risk framework there is a need for flexibility. A single 'one-size-fits all' framework is not a realistic option. Frameworks might differ by therapeutic area and because of regional differences such as patient characteristics and standards of care. The benefit–risk threshold can be affected by the seriousness of the condition being treated and the availability of other proven treatments. Flexibility is also needed because individuals differ from one another in how they perceive and value specific benefits and specific risks, for example the value of improved symptoms or the impact on survival. Account must also be taken of the fact that benefits and risks are not always measured by variables of comparable clinical significance thus limiting the ability to make direct comparisons without the use of appropriate weightings. Therefore, development of a benefit–risk framework should be cognisant of the influences of the decision-making process:

- a products benefit risk profile evolves through its life cycle

- benefit–risk decision making is one of the most critical activities in which stakeholders engage

- benefit–risk decisions have a significant impact on the products to which patients will have access and on how such products will be used

- critical activities are addressed by code or codes, for example 'good decision-making practice' (CMR International Institute Workshop, Victor Raczkowski 2008).

Current and future approaches to benefit–risk assessment for regulatory agencies – the FDA perspective

At the CMR International Institute Workshop (2008), Joyce Korvick from the FDA stated that the revised FDA mission statement is now expressed in terms of 'protecting' and 'advancing' public health by helping to speed innovations and helping to ensure that 'accurate, science-based information' is available not only to experts but to the people.

The assessment of benefit and risk for medicines, through a sound framework is integral to this mission. The analogy of the framework is for a bridge that links the 'benefit' data of the integrated summary of efficacy (ISE) to the 'risk' data in the integrated safety summary (ISS) – see Figure 6.1.

One weakness is that there is not currently a formal part of the regulatory submission for a discussion of the benefit–risk balance. There are possibilities for such discussion at the PSUR (Periodic Safety Update Report) stage but a framework is needed that applies to both the application and the review. This needs to be applicable throughout the product lifecycle, pre- and post-marketing as benefits and risks are dynamic and change with use and patient exposure to the product.

Factors in the discussion of such a framework include risk management plans, the availability of therapeutic options, and the ability to communicate the facts and uncertainties to populations and individual patients. Historically, the focus of clinical

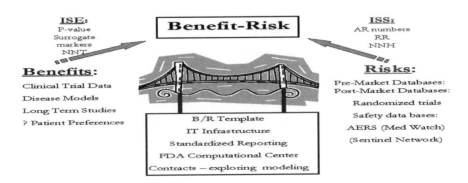

Figure 6.1 Bridging integrated summary of efficacy and safety (Reproduced from Joyce Korvick 2008)

development has been on establishing efficacy and clinical end points but there is not the same certainty, at the marketing stage in respect of safety and rare adverse events.

'Benefit–risk assessment has been largely limited to the presentation of the trial results without a summary of composite effect of both benefit and risk' and that the agency relies on 'enumerating the number and kinds of harms observed in trials'. In discussing the techniques and methodologies for evaluating benefit–risk there was a need to strike the right balance between over-complicated modelling and over simplicity, as well as concerns that models may give a 'false sense of precision'. A second issue was the communication of information in a transparent manner to a public that does not generally understand the benefit–risk 'tradeoffs' that need to be adopted when a medicine is approved. (Janet Woodcock, personal communication).

To move from a predominantly qualitative approach to benefit–risk assessment to a more quantitative approach is a major challenge, recognizing that the elements of benefits (efficacy) and risks (harms) are 'asymmetric': benefits are ascertained and reported differently from harms in randomized controlled trials (RCTs). Such trials are sized to detect differences in defined efficacy endpoints but analytical approaches to safety are relatively unsophisticated.

The current integration of benefit and risk evaluation is qualitative and ways to move forward include improving the transparency of the decision-making process throughout the life cycle of drugs and biologic products. This includes communication of benefits and risks to healthcare providers and patients based upon timely assessments. Thus, framework development is necessary to the evolving approaches to benefit–risk assessment and the move towards a more quantitative model for decision-making and analysis (CMR International Institute for Regulatory Science Workshop, Joyce Korvick 2008). For example the following represents some of the advantages and shortcomings of the more recent approaches (models) to benefit–risk assessment.

Advantages

- enhance consistency and comprehensiveness in the process of expressing the benefit–risk balance;

- enhance transparency of regulatory decisions

- force assessors to focus on benefit–risk

- provide a tool to compare products in relation to the MCDA model, the usefulness of the sensitivity analysis was particularly recognized.

Shortcomings

- does not enhance objectivity of benefit–risk decision-making (the numerical outcome of the analysis from the model may give a false reassurance)

- deviation between the outcome from the model and the regulators' final decision would be difficult to explain

- building a model for every situation and factor, with discussions on values and weightings is time-consuming and may require more time/resources than are available

- there are potential conflicts between industry and regulators in the way in which a product is scored.

Quantitative assessment of clinical benefit–risk at FDA: what needs to change and how to move forward?

At the CMR International Institute for Regulatory Science Workshop, Bob O'Neill (FDA) gave his perspective on the RCTs, which are primarily designed to demonstrate efficacy with the science of quantifying risks and harms lagging behind. This imbalance must be addressed and new assessment tools need to be developed if a workable benefit–risk framework is to be achieved.

There are differences in the way safety data are evaluated from a quantitative aspect and different approaches to adverse events are needed when considering, for example, treatment versus prevention, acute versus chronic exposure/usage and severity and frequency/rarity of the condition. Data on risks can derive from RCTs but can be external to these, often from spontaneous reporting and observational databases within health care plans such as Medicare and Medicaid in the United States. The benefit–risk balance is a function of time that will change over the life-cycle of the product in the market place where one is dealing with a multiplicity of benefits, risks and competing events.

Three situations exist: first, where benefits and risks of a new molecular entity are observed only in RCTs and evaluations are based primarily on these; second, where the benefits are observed in clinical trials but potential risks are observed outside of the trials and are not quantifiable; and third, where benefits and risk change over time, with multiple usage, and emerging information. Thus, development of a benefit–risk framework must take account of these situations which informs the regulators of benefit–risk decisions. In this context issues relevant to establishing the framework include:

- metrics of benefits
- metrics of harm (risks)
- metrics of benefit and risk considered jointly
- benefit–risk assessment as a function of exposure time
- population versus individual patient benefit–risk
- benefit–risk assessment at time of approval versus life cycle
- role of RCTs in the estimation of benefits and risks.

As noted, RCTs are primarily designed to evaluate efficacy rather than safety, as a result of which:

- safety endpoints may not be as precisely measured or adjudicated as in efficacy trials where there are a few pre-specified endpoints

- exposure time may be critical to onset of events (dose, cumulative dose, mechanism of action, liver damage)

- safety events can occur after withdrawal from exposure – lack of follow-up in a study can lead to loss of this information

- there may be recurrent events and multiple different events per subject

- the way in which events are counted and coded, even under the agreed Medical Dictionary for Regulatory Activities (MedDRA) terminology, might not be consistent and uniformly applied.

The consequences are that safety endpoints are measured, collected, or followed with less accuracy than for efficacy and 'after the fact' the endpoints may get adjudicated, when it is too late to obtain other patient information that may be pertinent to the adjudication. This asymmetry needs to be addressed if the net benefits are to be better quantified, in particular, the detection of delayed and late onset side effects that will be missed through inadequate follow-up, especially of patients that withdraw from trials.

The CONSORT (Consolidated Standards of Reporting Trials) checklist for reporting clinical trials was drawn up by a group of journal editors and scientists and first published in 1996. Although subsequently modified, the 22-item list, in 2003, included only one point that was specifically addressed to safety. In response to concerns about the reporting of harms in RCTs, the CONSORT Statement was revised to include 10 new items about reporting harms-related issues.

Although there is an internationally agreed ICH guideline on *The Structure and Content of Clinical Study Reports* (ICH E3, 1996a), the FDA clinical reviewers look at the raw data beneath these summary reports and study the line-listings for individual patients. FDA publishes a 102-page internal *Reviewer Guidance* for 'Conducting a Clinical Safety Review of a New Product Application and Preparing a Report on the Review'. It is an intricate and complicated process currently requiring physical cross-checking of line-listings in printouts and there is scope for a fundamental overhaul of the way the large volumes of data are submitted electronically for review. Analytical tools are needed that will display the data visually at a patient level as well as conceptualizing time dependencies (cumulative exposure, interaction with other medications, covariates).

The FDA Computational Center is exploring the use of available electronic tools and possibilities for developing new ones. Potential approaches include:

- visual graphics and informative displays giving individual subject case report profiles

- summarizing patient outcomes by treatment group

- comparisons of treatment groups with respect to patterns and event rates (events history charts)

- new measures of cumulative events - counting events and adjusting for duration of exposure.

Strategies for exploring associations, multiplicities, time dependencies, syndromes, event combinations, etc., depend heavily on the integrity of the coding of adverse events using MedDRA. Companies using several Contract Research Organizations for clinical trials often overlook the importance of coordinating and monitoring a uniform coding strategy. It is therefore essential that companies allocate time in planning their Investigational New Drug/New Drug Approvals (IND/NDA) process to discuss with FDA prospective plans for the collection and analysis of safety outcomes.

Appropriate quantification of benefit and risk is just beginning to be understood and addressed. There is a need to borrow from other epidemiological fields and understand better the limits and practicalities of quantifying efficacy and harms. Quantification of efficacy is more refined with 30 years of development and guidelines but the quantification of safety (risk, harm) is far behind. Hence, the thesis exists that there is currently an asymmetry in benefit–risk quantification. To this end, a prerequisite of a framework for benefit–risk assessment is that the scientific level for both safety and efficacy must be comparable and this will require work on standards for clinical trials, data formats and tools for access, storage and retrieval.

Finally, a culture change is needed to recognize that new tools and new approaches must be adopted, for example to recognize that epidemiological observational studies are no substitute for large trials from which low-level signals can be quantified. Furthermore, the talent base and training are not currently in place that would allow a true understanding of the science of safety assessment and the science of evaluating benefit and risk (CMR International Institute for Regulatory Science Workshop, Bob O'Neill, 2008).

A Health Canada perspective

Health Canada initiated, in the fourth quarter of 2006, a third major evolution of its regulatory framework through amendments to the Food and Drugs Act and its Regulations, processes and practices (CMR International Institute for Regulatory Science Workshop, Robyn Lim, 2008). The principles of the Progressive Licensing Project (PLP) can be summarized as an evidence-based and life-cycle approach backed by health outcomes; good planning and accountability. The PLP provides an

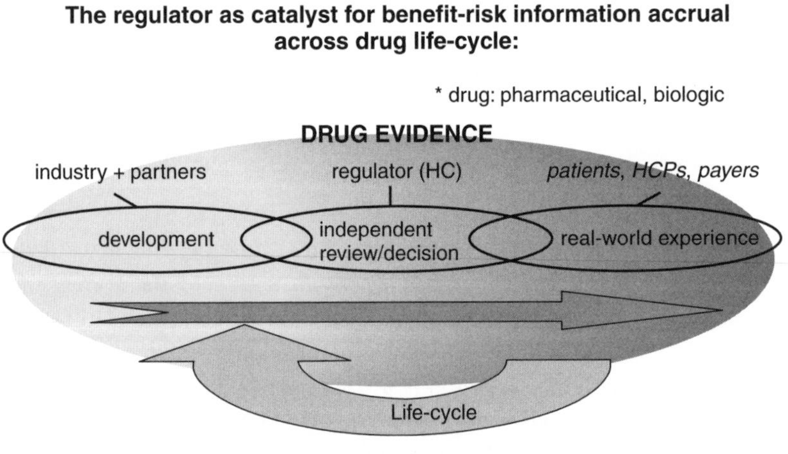

The regulator as catalyst for benefit-risk information accrual across drug life-cycle:

Figure 6.2 The regulator as a catalyst for benefit–risk information accrual across drug life-cycle (Reproduced from Robyn Lim 2008)

opportunity to ensure that appropriate benefit–risk assessment considerations are included in the drug regulatory framework through best practices.

The regulator can be seen as a 'catalyst' to direct, support, encourage best evidence, methodologies and practices in benefit–risk consideration. Although the primary, visible, role of the regulator is at the review and decision-making stage, they can also form a link throughout the evidence chain from development by industry and its partners to the 'real world' decisions made by patients, healthcare professionals and payers (see Figure 6.2).

At the workshop in 2008 Robyn Lim stated that whilst the core, primary data for a benefit–risk assessment are safety, efficacy and quality (SEQ), the concept is much broader. 'Secondary' and 'tertiary' layers of evidence can be identified that are implicit but are important drivers for regulatory decisions.

Secondary levels of evidence can be considered as 'performance framing' and reflect the conditions of use, impact and utility of the product and include:

- the nature of disease/condition (e.g. life-threatening versus non-debilitating)

- the nature of the drug's effect on the disease/condition (e.g. disease modifying versus symptomatic management)

- the nature of the target population (e.g. vulnerable populations, level of overall health, degree of heterogeneity)

- the nature of the treatment environment (e.g. availability, performance, uncertainties of other therapies) and the degree of unmet medical need

- clinical practice environments (domestic, international) and the clinical expectations for the product

- practicality issues, including anticipated compliance, convenience of use, anticipated risk manageability

- anticipated use patterns once on market, which may lie outside the conditions of use studied and approved.

Tertiary levels of evidence are considerations that go beyond specific drug performance and include such issues as:

- population *versus* more individualized health considerations

- access issues ('choice' and 'hope')

- the risk tolerance and uncertainty tolerance of decision makers

- the ability to accrue further SEQ evidence after approval and marketing, e.g. the ethical and logistical challenges of enrolling patients into further trials.

Regulatory benefit–risk assessment can be viewed as a context analysis, a gap analysis and an options analysis. As a *context analysis* benefit–risk assessment can be seen as adding layers upon the SEQ evidence, allowing for considerations of conditions of use that are necessary for decisions to be realistic and relevant in the 'real-world'. It has a broader scope than the SEQ analysis and is often less systematic and more qualitative as it incorporates values and ethics as well as the perspectives and perceived roles of industry, payers, healthcare practitioners and patients. benefit–risk assessment is a *gap analysis* in that it needs to bridge the 'uncertainty gap' between the pre-market review and the 'real world' conditions of use. The benefit–risk assessment as an *options analysis* can provide a management strategy for optimizing benefits and minimizing risks through the conditions of licensing, risk management plans and appropriate labelling. Visual benefit–risk assessment tools, including graphical and pictorial representations of benefit–risk balance, are currently under development at Health Canada to support reviewers' best practices and regulatory decision-making transparency.

The benefit–risk assessment of medicines aligns with Canada's federal framework for science-based decision making about risk which is based on the application of precaution but recognizes the necessity for decision making in the face of a lack of full scientific certainty about risks. The range of tools for precautionary measures include measures to manage and/or reduce drug uncertainties and it is recognized that a simple accept/reject decisions can stall evidence development and identification of risks and benefits.

The overarching element of benefit–risk assessment, however, is judgement and comprehensive benefit–risk assessment reveals the necessity for judgement calls more explicitly than SEQ assessment. Judgement is required regarding the interpretation of the extent and meaning of the evidence available and the uncertainties in the SEQ and benefit–risk evidence that will always exist (Robyn Lim 2008).

CHMP perspective

At the CMR International Institute for Regulatory Science Workshop (2008), Professor Flamion (Chair, Scientific Advice Working Party EMEA) described a new project at the CHMP which had produced a number of recommendations (reference CHMP Reflection Paper – March 2008 – see Appendix 3).

- First, there should be a revision of the current benefit–risk assessment section of the final CHMP Assessment Report template (Appendix 3), incorporating a structured list of benefit–risk criteria with appropriate guidance

- Second, the CHMP should conduct further research into the methodology of benefit–risk assessment, involving further experts and assessors.

Development of a benefit–risk assessment template should:

- use a structured and mainly qualitative approach

- describe sources of uncertainty and variability and their impact on the benefit–risk assessment

- indicate the amount and accuracy of available evidence

- be explicit about the perspectives of the various stakeholders, in particular patients and treating physicians

- define the level of risk acceptability corresponding to the perceived degree of clinical benefit (in the specific context)

- state the benefits in a way that is comparable to risks (e.g. NNT/NNH) – avoid relative expressions of benefit and risk

- describe how the benefit–risk balance may vary across different factors (e.g. patient characteristics)

- discuss the sensitivity of the benefit–risk balance assessment to different assumptions. regular training and monitoring should also be put in place.

Development and testing of new tools should:

- describe the current practice of benefit–risk assessment in the EU regulatory network

- examine the applicability of current models, tools and processes, assessed against criteria relevant for benefit–risk assessment at different stages of drug development/approval

- field test selected models/tools (in one or more domains)

- develop a new method to be used as a decision-aid for benefit–risk assessment by regulators

- develop a training package for assessors.

6.3 PREREQUISITES OF A BENEFIT–RISK FRAMEWORK FOR THE REGISTRATION OF A NEW MEDICINE

It is generally acknowledged that there are no 'safe' medicines and the possibilities of harms are accepted in return for possible benefits that outweigh them. There appears, however, to be a greater emphasis on risk, for example in risk management plans, than on benefits. Whilst a formal framework for risk management has been in existence for several years (with a cursory mention of benefit the context of balancing benefit–risk) there are no regulatory standards for benefit–risk evaluation or guidance on how to carry it out. The current approach can appear to be a 'black box' within which decisions are made using a 'heuristic' approach of learning by experience (CMR International Institute for Regulatory Science Workshop, John Ferguson 2008).

Whilst a heuristic approach continues to have its place, without transparency and structure the benefits of such learnings are lost, especially as complexity increases. Furthermore, without a standardized framework for integrating and weighting the evidence, the process becomes inscrutable, subjective and piece-meal. The regulatory implications of subjectiveness and reliance on individual judgement can be that different decisions are made and different actions taken within and between agencies.

A survey, which included US, European and Japanese pharma/biotech companies and two European regulatory agencies, was carried out and reported to the DIA Annual Conference, Boston, 2008 (Whitebrook and Markey, 2008). The results indicated a high level of interest in a structured framework for balancing benefit and risk but indicated that the current emphasis is on risk management plans with the emphasis on risk. A small proportion of companies are actively investigating or using structured benefit–risk approaches and a still smaller number investigating the use of quantitative measures.

In accepting the value of a framework or other models it must be acknowledged that these are decision aids and not statements of scientific fact. Figure 6.3 sets out the benefits of a benefit–risk framework and the by-products that can be expected to accrue (CMR International Institute for Regulatory Science Workshop, John Ferguson, 2008).

Value of a BR Framework

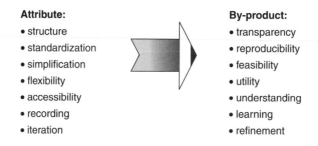

Attribute:
- structure
- standardization
- simplification
- flexibility
- accessibility
- recording
- iteration

By-product:
- transparency
- reproducibility
- feasibility
- utility
- understanding
- learning
- refinement

Figure 6.3 Value of a benefit–risk framework (Reproduced from John Ferguson 2008)

The prerequisites for a workable framework include the need to:

- adapt to any indication
- capture and address perceptions of multiple stakeholders
- be accessible to all stakeholders
- weigh/prioritize all available data
- capture variability and uncertainty
- allow for time-dependence
- support balancing on a common scale
- support cross-product comparisons
- have acceptable operating characteristics
- support registration and labelling.

The pharmaceutical industry is working on a structured benefit–risk framework that has as its two main components: a value tree and data tables. The framework defines the way in which the elements from the data tables are to be associated with the value tree and the weightings that should be assigned to these elements. Further work is required on the development of such a framework but the basic design has been informed by consultation with academics and regulators as well as modelling and risk management experts. A test bed has been developed and funding has been secured to start testing this using actual but 'anonymized' products and by adding simulated data to extend the framework or model as far as possible.

As indicated in Figure 6.4, decision frameworks have a role in all types of decision-making but quantitative models are likely to become increasingly important as the

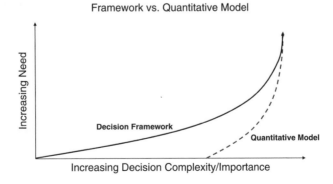

Figure 6.4 Need for structure in decision making (Reproduced from John Ferguson 2008)

complexity increases. Quantitative models should therefore be incorporated in frameworks that are specifically designed to accommodate them. A framework can therefore be seen as the basis for specifying desirable, context-specific model characteristics and setting performance requirements (validation) for quantitative (mathematical) models (CMR International Institute for Regulatory Science Workshop, John Ferguson 2008).

Remembering that decision models are *aids* to decision making and not statements of scientific fact, and conclusions derived from them will be conditional on the assumptions that are made. Structural assumptions must, therefore, be explicitly reported and these assumptions along with parameter estimates must be assessed against the data. The dependency of the output upon input data should be tested using sensitivity analysis. Furthermore, patient preferences are an important factor that requires further evaluation in relation to the ways they can be used as an adjunct to frameworks and quantitative models in order to inform thinking.

Ultimately, benefit risk assessment is about the patient and the prescriber. There must be a shared understanding of decision making and decisions through a structured framework and no 'black box' decision aids.

Only decision-making processes based on the pursuit of negotiated outcomes, conducted in an open and transparent manner and inclusive of all legitimate actors involved in the issue are likely to resolve the complex issues surrounding the balancing of benefits and risk for pharmaceuticals, biologics and vaccines (modified from the World Commission on Dams Report, 2000).

6.4 CURRENT STATUS OF BENEFIT–RISK ASSESSMENT AMONG COMPANIES AND AGENCIES

Neil McAuslane (Director of Institute for Regulatory Science) described a survey carried out in 2008 to assess the current status of benefit–risk assessment among companies and agencies (CMR International Institute for Regulatory Science Workshop, Neil McAuslane 2008). This was as a follow up to the earlier survey described in chapter 2, a brief survey was carried out with the following objectives namely to:

- identify companies' and agencies' current approaches to benefit–risk assessment and investigate current perceptions of the models/frameworks available or being developed

- identify the parameters that need to be included in a framework for measuring benefit–risk in order to make the framework fit for purpose.

The survey questionnaire was sent to the 23 companies and to 13 regulatory agencies: EMEA and six EU national agencies; US FDA (CDER and CBER); Health Canada; TGA,

Australia; Swissmedic, Switzerland; and HSA, Singapore. Responses were received from 9 companies and 10 agencies. The topics covered in the questionnaire included:

- types and timing of the benefit–risk assessment currently used by the agency/company

- parameters taken into account to assess benefit–risk

- perception of the need for an appropriate benefit–risk framework

- views on the value of published models/frameworks for benefit–risk assessment

- the major hurdles and possible solutions when looking at a possible benefit–risk framework.

Quantitative and qualitative methods

The response to whether their system for benefit–risk assessment system for pre-submission was quantitative *versus* qualitative is shown in Table 6.1.

Table 6.1 Quantitative and qualitative methods of benefit–risk assessment currently used by companies and agencies

Statement	Companies	Agencies
Qualitative Our internal system is a purely qualitative system based on internal experts or management making a 'gut decision' on the benefit–risk profile of each product	4/9	6/10[a]
Semiquantitative Our internal system is semiquantitative in that it has a structured (written) framework or standard operating procedure for data collection and analysis but also incorporates expert judgement into the final decision	4/9	4/10[a]
Quantitative Our internal system is a fully quantitative model, which gives a benefit–risk ratio for a new medicine. Experts and management simply oversee and approve the results	1/9[b]	0/10

[a] One agency answered positively for both qualitative and semiqualitative.
[b] The company indicating that its assessment was fully quantitative puts a value on each of the benefit and risk parameters and these are weighted.

Stage of benefit –risk assessment

Respondents were asked about the stage at which they use a benefit–risk assessment as part of the decision-making process and the responses are shown in Figure 6.5.

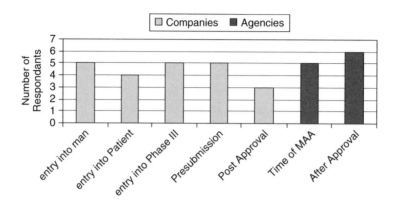

Figure 6.5 Stage of benefit–risk assessment by companies and agencies (Reproduced from Neil McAuslane 2008)

The results indicated that companies are using benefit–risk assessments throughout the pre-submission development stage but, as might be expected, only 3/5 reported that they used the same assessment system at all stages.

Agencies reported using benefit–risk assessment both before and after approval and 3/6 use the same system at both stages. Five of the 9 companies and 4 of the 10 agencies reported that they used a model (CMR International Institute for Regulatory Science Workshop, Neil McAuslane 2008).

Parameters for assessing benefit risk

The questionnaire included a list of safety and efficacy parameters that might be used to evaluate benefit and risk and a list of parameters relevant to assessing the benefit–risk ratio or balance when making the assessment. Companies and agencies were not only asked which they used for their own procedures but also to give a view on whether they should be included in a formal benefit–risk framework with wider applicability. Other parameters that were reported as being used in current systems are shown in Table 6.2.

The need for a benefit–risk framework

The questionnaire included 15 statements relating to the need for, and usefulness of, developing a formal benefit–risk framework that might have a wider use outside individual companies and agencies. Respondents were asked to rate the statements from

Table 6.2 Additional benefit–risk parameters reported by the companies and agencies

Safety	Efficacy	Benefit–risk balance
Adverse effects of other therapies for the indication	Validation of outcome measure	Risk management programmes beneficial
Manageability/practicality of options	Minimally effective dose	[a]Seriousness of the medical condition
Dose–response effects	Comparison with other therapies	[a]Availability of other proven therapies (or lack thereof)
AE impact on disease context	Standard of care	
Possible linkage between AE	Relevance to domestic population (local practice issues and disease epidemiology)	
Anticipated population AEs	Long-term effect	
Relevance to domestic population	Waning of effect	
Dependence	Availability of alternatives	
Reversibility	Relative efficacy	
Transmission of AE to close contacts (live vaccine virus)	Dosing duration needed	
Relative safety with other products with same indication	Advantages with dosage forms	
Vulnerability of the population (infants versus adults)	Population benefiting	
Preventability of AE	Conditions of use (pandemic, terrorist attack)	
Risk period (risk only when being administered or does risk persist beyond administration)	[a]Convenience factor (e.g. storage, acquisition, monitoring, etc.)	
[a]Safety profile compared to standard treatment and medical need	[a]Importance of considering lowest effective dose	
[a]Robustness of safety results		
[a]Laboratory data (particularly liver, renal and muscle enzymes)		

AE, adverse event.
[a] Company responses.
Source: Neil McAuslane, 2008.

'Strongly agree' to Strongly disagree'. The results, showing the percentage of agencies and companies that responded 'strongly agree' or 'agree' are summarized in Table 6.3.

Use of published models

The questionnaire identified three specific, established models for assessing benefits and risk: The 'Principle of Threes', the 'Turbo Model' and MCDA. Respondents were

Table 6.3   The need for a benefit–risk framework

Statement	Agency A %	Company C %	Diff
The purpose of establishing an appropriate benefit–risk framework is to improve:			
1. The consistency of decision making	100	100	0
2. The transparency of decision making	100	100	0
3. Communication of the decision	100	100	0
There is a need for a benefit–risk framework to be developed that can be used by both agencies and companies	90	100	10
It is important that any benefit–risk framework, if developed for registration purposes is utilized across regulatory divisions within an agency and across agencies worldwide	89	67	22
This benefit–risk framework should also be applicable to health technology assessment groups	75	89	−14
An appropriate benefit–risk framework for registration should also enable assessment of risk management plans	70	89	−19
It is important that all stakeholders (agencies, companies, doctors and patients) are part of the development and validation of an appropriate benefit–risk framework	70	89	−19
For the registration of new medicinal products it will be possible to develop an overarching benefit–risk framework	67	100	−33
An appropriate benefit–risk framework for registration should also apply to all stages of drug development from cradle to grave	60	67	−7
Our company/agency preference would be a quantitative approach to benefit–risk assessment rather than a purely qualitative approach	56	63	−7
For the registration of new medicinal products it will be necessary to develop therapeutic area specific benefit–risk frameworks	50	67	−17
The best framework for benefit–risk assessment would be a decision tree approach	25	63	−38
The purpose of an appropriate benefit–risk framework is to define a number that translates the benefit–risk ratio in absolute terms and can be used to measure its sensitivity to various parameters	22	38	−16

Key: Diff = A% − C%.
Source: Neil McAuslane 2008.

asked for their knowledge and opinion of these rated from 'highly valuable' to 'barely relevant'. Respondents also indicated where they had no knowledge of the system. The results are shown in Figure 6.6.

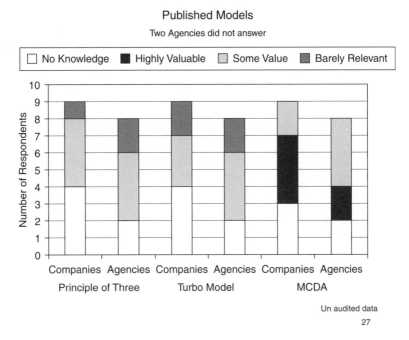

Figure 6.6   Use of published models by the companies and agencies (Reproduced from CMR International Institute for Regulatory Science 2008)

As shown, only the MCDA model scored as a 'highly valuable' model among both companies and agencies. Three agencies and 4 companies referred to other published frameworks or models currently available. These included: benefit–risk profiling; patient preferences; quality of life (QALY); incremental net benefit; and NNT/NNH. Reference was also made to the EMEA/CHMP Reflection paper (Appendix 4).

Barriers and solutions

In the survey, participants were asked to give views on the barriers (top three major hurdles) to achieving a benefit–risk framework that could have 'universal' application and possible solutions to overcome these hurdles. Responses generally fell into three categories:

- issues relating to stakeholders, particularly patients
- quantifying benefit and risk
- models and acceptance.

Table 6.4   Barriers and solutions to achieving benefit–risk framework[a]

Major hurdles	Possible solutions
Issues relating to stakeholders, particularly the patient	
Patients differ in how they value specific benefits and value specific risks	Allow for flexibility in pharmaceutical development plans and in regulatory decision making to avoid a 'one size fits all' approach
Patients differ in how they perceive specific benefits and perceive specific risks	Allow for flexibility in pharmaceutical development plans and in regulatory decision making to avoid a 'one size fits all' approach
Communicating and defining value judgements and risks	More education of patients and patient groups
Communication tools to explain to researchers, regulators, prescribers and patients how a benefit–risk assessment is done and how to interpret it	Multi-stakeholder working groups to develop appropriate, state-of-the-art tools
In the context of achieving an appropriate benefit–risk framework that is universally usable by all stakeholders, one of the major difficulties would be the inherent differences in the systems and risks among the stakeholders; unless the Framework is otherwise sufficiently generic such that it can be adopted and developed further according to the needs of the individual agency/company	
Quantifying benefit and risk	
Benefits and risks are measured in clinical studies in ways than are difficult to compare directly (i.e. 'apples and pears')	When applicable and feasible, measure benefits and risks with measures that can be compared with one another
How to quantify risks and benefits on some common scale. What that common scale should be is controversial	Assessments need to be made consistently. One would want to know if the decision is sensitive to the choice of scale (e.g. NNT versus NNH; QALYs, etc.); the point is that the relative values are important when making therapeutic choices, even if the absolute values are not easily interpretable
Uncertainty in data from random variation, unclear causality, or	Better data collection instruments, larger studies, more targeted
Subgroup heterogeneity	Patient pools. Multi-stakeholder working groups to develop appropriate, state-of-the-art approaches
General agreement on specific values for each criterion	Agreement could be reached through meetings but this is highly time-consuming

A point that bothers people is the 'tyranny of the average', that is, the benefit: risk discussion, they argue, should be made on an individual patient basis. This does NOT reduce the value of quantification, but does argue in favour of providing a *range* of benefit: risk values for various assumptions about the importance placed on specific items, whether benefits or risks, by individual patients

We may never agree on a single value of NNT/NNH or any other measure that can serve as a universal threshold, but a threshold might be defined for an individual patient or a homogeneous group of patients. We will certainly never agree on specific 'weights' (utilities, etc.) to assign that would apply to all patients

What 'benefits' should be counted? Should 'convenience' factors matter, for example? Patient reported outcomes (PRO's) should certainly matter, but it's hard to meet FDA standards for how to study those

Broader inclusion of a range of 'benefits', with varying weights or importance assigned to those benefits. Convenience (or some other attribute) may not matter to the agency, but may matter a *lot* to patients

Comparative efficacy and safety data against Standard of Care, especially where head-to-head trials would require enormous size to achieve adequate statistical power

Not sure

Models and acceptance

Concern that these frameworks minimize the importance of clinical judgement and decision making

Identify methods that have their foundation in clinical judgement while offering transparency and consistency in application of such judgement

Entrenched views tend to 'bang the drum' for a particular framework

Industry/academia/agencies partnership to review and validate methodologies

Lack of pragmatism – *the perfect is the enemy of the good*

Continue to highlight how many criticisms being raised re: possible solutions in this area actually already exist today one of the biggest gains is transparency and consistency in decision making

Lack of institutional experience, expertise, and resources to implement

More public discussions like this one; development of training

Use of new frameworks

Programmes in the field

Preparation of disease models on indications models

Test different systems-methods on real life data

Lack of globally harmonized regulatory approach

ICH-like harmonization

Lack of common inter-company approach

Regulatory harmonization

No single commonly accepted methodology

None at this time

Complexity of the decision process

The model needs sophistication yet should be easily comprehensible

---

[a] Compilation (verbatim) of the responses received from the companies and regulators.
Source: CMR International Institute for Regulatory Science Workshop Report, Neil McAuslane, 2008.

6.5   CONSTRUCTING A BENEFIT–RISK FRAMEWORK

Essential elements for a benefit–risk framework

The feasibility of establishing the basis for a universally applicable benefit–risk framework that would be of value to both regulatory agencies and companies is now a priority. The first step towards this goal has been established by reviewing and proposing a list of parameters to be included in the benefit–risk assessment of a new medicine but more work is needed to develop this further. In summary:

- agreement is needed on a common terminology or 'lexicon' to avoid ambiguity in discussions

- regulatory agencies from the 'emerging nations' should be included as well as established authorities early on in the further development of the framework.

Taking forward the benefit–risk framework

At the CMR International Institute for Regulatory Science Workshop in 2008, the following recommendations were made for specific studies to be undertaken:

- a pilot project including case studies to test the framework among different stakeholders (patients, physicians, companies and regulators)

- a comparative study of current regulatory review templates relating to benefit–risk analysis, with a view to improving the consistency and value of the assessment

- further development of the framework should include considerations that might also be applicable to the Health Technology Assessment (HTA) of the product for reimbursement.

Managing benefit and risk throughout the product lifecycle

It is envisaged that any future approach should look at the way in which the benefit–risk framework could be applied at different stages in the lifecycle of new medicine and integrated into risk management plans (RMPs). Any such system should take into account specific points listed below:

- ensuring that the patient perspective was taken into account when considering RMPs

- examining the challenges of using electronic databases versus other methods for obtaining follow-up information on the safety and use of approved products

- using case studies to illustrate benefit–risk profiling throughout a product's life cycle.

The benefit–risk framework should be seen as a positive advance for tracking the evolution of benefit and risk information throughout the lifecycle of a product. The concept of managing the benefit–risk profile up to and beyond product approval should be incorporated in a future benefit–risk framework with the focus on integrating benefit–risk assessment into risk management plans. In such context, the patient perspective should also be included.

The future framework for benefit–risk appraisal of medicines should focus specifically on continuing benefit–risk assessments into the post-approval phase, but should capture the way the benefit–risk profile impacts all stages of development. A diagrammatic representation of the ways in which benefit–risk considerations are embedded in the different stages of development is given in Figure 6.7. The correct application of benefit–risk analyses at the critical decision stages (e.g. discovery to development and

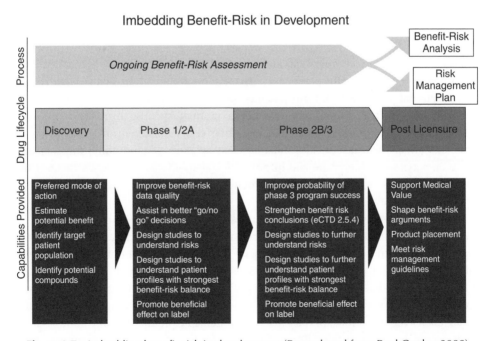

Figure 6.7 Imbedding benefit-risk in development (Reproduced from Paul Coplan 2008)

end of Phase II) could inform the scale and direction of the subsequent development programme in a way that would soon justify the additional investment (time and additional statistical/epidemiological resources).

Communicating benefit and risk to stakeholders

The framework initiative should address the difficult issues that are constantly faced by both agencies and companies in trying to explain to key stakeholders the methodology and outcomes of benefit–risk assessment that may affect the availability and use of the new medicines. Such a process can be better facilitated by consideration of all three or any of the following:

- establishing current communication practices among companies and regulatory agencies

- ensuring that issues were discussed with all relevant stakeholders: patients, physicians, pharmacists and the media

- developing methods with which to assess *communication strategies* and the need for *general education* on the meaning of, and methodologies for, benefit–risk assessments.

This is recognized as a complex and multi-layered issue that could be approached from many angles according to the perceived purpose of communication, that is, whether it is an educational exercise to inform patients, physicians and the public of the way in which benefit–risk decisions are made or a product specific exercise to provide information on a particular medicine, including crisis management when potential problems arise. Pharmaceutical companies and agencies should come together and agree on ways to both educate and inform key stakeholders on the assessment of the benefits and risks of medicines with particular reference to the development of the benefit–risk framework.

In addition, it would be necessary to set a research agenda to assemble information on the current situation. A literature review that went beyond communication on healthcare issues and included a broader review of social science would be useful. An objective of this review would be to gain a better understanding of perceptions of benefit and risk by different stakeholders. Furthermore, a survey should be conducted to look at current communication practices that are in place, or have been used by companies and regulatory agencies for educational purposes or to communicate product-specific issues. Such a study would be useful in identifying, for example, whether there are communication practices that are targeted differently to different patient groups and/or stakeholders. Additionally, the value of patient information leaflets could be assessed in such survey.

The proposed study could incorporate a gap analysis between patients' needs for benefit–risk information and the approach being taken by industry and authorities. This would, however, require sources of information on perceived patients'/carers' feedback on timing, format and content of such information.

The survey would need to include respondents representing stakeholders other than industry and agencies: patients, physicians, pharmacists and the media. The issues to be considered in the survey should include:

- the effectiveness of communication strategies and different forms of communication practices

- identification of target audiences (e.g. sufferers from chronic diseases versus acute illness, experienced patient groups versus newcomers)

- support for physicians and pharmacists in their communication with their patients to ensure consistency in the messages given

- case studies that illustrate the way sensitive issues have been addressed, including those where there have been conflicting views between regulators and sponsors.

In addition, the following topics also need to be addressed.

- Regulatory decisions and conditions – the role and usefulness of current information from regulatory agencies, e.g. the EU 'triumvirate' of EPAR, product information (label) and patient information leaflet (PIL).

- Crisis communications – the effectiveness of different approaches when urgent issues arise and the need to look beyond the 'reactive' response to possibilities for proactive communication strategies.

- Patient compliance – the role of communication in improving the way in which patients take medicines and adhere to instructions should be covered. It should also be remembered that with increased patient empowerment individuals can influence the choice of medicines. Input might also be sought from the Medicines Use Review (MUR) among pharmacists in the UK.

Communications strategy

Strategies adopted by agencies and pharmaceutical companies might include the establishment of communications divisions, procedures for press briefings and cooperation with patient support groups. A few examples of such strategies are highlighted below.

- Internal communication – it is equally important to ensure good communications within companies/agencies to ensure a consistent and credible approach.

- Educational role – communications can have an educational role in preparing stakeholders to receive and understand benefit–risk messages in addition to making them receptive to product-specific information.

- Handling the media – developing strategies for countering the 'negative' messages and images about medicines often portrayed in the press.

- Measuring effectiveness determining whether agencies and companies are taking steps to measure the impact of communication strategies or carrying out benchmarking exercises.

Towards a universal framework – a global approach

A common foundation for benefit–risk assessment needs to be defined that would be applicable across different company and agency platforms and different geographical regions. A common framework of the elements to be considered routinely would benefit both regulators and sponsors. Companies would be able to design their R&D programmes to ensure that the relevant data items are covered in the regulatory dossier (CMR International Institute for Regulatory Science Workshop Report, 2008).

The 'default' primary audience is the labelled population for the medicine but there will be cases where public health issues need to be taken into account; the assessment should extend beyond the patient level to the population level. Also, the benefit–risk assessment might differ if looked at from the patient/physician perspective rather than a regulatory perspective based on efficacy and primary endpoints.

A universal framework for benefit–risk assessment should be able to accommodate changes in the benefit–risk balance. It also must not focus only on the data that is applicable at the pre-approval and post-launch stages. Benefit–risk assessment must be seen as a continuum that needs to be revisited throughout the product life-cycle, taking account of post-marketing surveillance and epidemiological data. To this effect surrogate endpoints should be confirmed in the post-marketing phase and will have an impact on the benefit–risk assessment. Furthermore, the therapeutic environment will change and it may be necessary to re-evaluate the benefits and risks between products including older, well-established products that may need to be re-assessed in the light of therapeutic advances.

A quantitative benefit–risk model would force discipline and accountability and would assist communication of risk. Practical problems in achieving this must, however be recognized especially in terms of agreeing on the basis for weighting the relative importance of different criteria, in the context of a product's use. Quantitative metrics that might derive from a standardised benefit–risk framework is not a substitute for decision making. The outcome of such a framework would help inform the assessment as judgement aid.

The adoption of a universal benefit–risk framework should not follow the 'traditional' pattern of development and acceptance by the established agencies (ICH regions, Canada, Australia) before being discussed with agencies in other regions. It must therefore be ensured that agencies representing the 'emerging' nations in the field of drug regulation are included, from the start, in formal moves towards the development of a basic framework for benefit–risk assessment. (Workshop report, 2008).

A common terminology

Different interpretations are often placed on different terms used to discuss benefit–risk even at the level of defining a 'benefit–risk framework' versus a 'benefit–risk model'. In taking the framework forward, work should start with the development of a lexicon to ensure common, defined use of terms. For example, benefit–risk ratio terminology, as 'traditionally' applied to benefit–risk evaluations, should be avoided as it implies that a definitive metric can be calculated for comparing benefit and risk. The terms 'benefit risk balance' or 'profile' may be more appropriate.

Enhancement of regulatory review templates

The CMR International Institute for Regulatory Science Workshop (2008) examined how regulatory review templates might incorporate the benefit–risk framework. It was agreed that there is a need to carry out a comparative study of current regulatory review templates with a view to improving the consistency and value of benefit–risk analyses. The objectives of the study would be to:

- compare the review templates currently being used by regulatory agencies and evaluate whether an overarching benefit–risk framework could enhance criteria for benefit–risk review, within the template

- increase the awareness of reviewers of the current discussions on benefit–risk models for evaluating value and risk

- encourage the application of a more consistent framework for benefit–risk review among different agencies.

Impact of benefit–risk framework on presentation of benefit–risk arguments in regulatory submission

The way in which companies present comparative efficacy and safety data in submission dossiers is often deficient. Would the benefit–risk framework improve this? Risks are not well identified in RCTs: Could trial design be improved through early benefit–risk analysis? Benefits are often overlooked in the post-approval phase when the emphasis is on risk detection. Would the balance be redressed by on-going benefit–risk evaluations? The 'geography' of risk detection has changed over the last 10 years. Although new medicines are often filed almost simultaneously in the EU and United States there is a 'reimbursement lag' before marketing in Europe with the result that post-approval detection of novel safety issues now occurs earlier in the United States. How does this impact the ongoing benefit–risk assessment? The addition of new indications later in the lifecycle provides an opportunity for extending the benefit–risk profile to a new patient population. Can the benefit–risk framework accommodate such changes?

Challenges in assessing benefit and risks in the post-approval phase

Data from electronic databases of patient records have been advocated as a means of tracking usage and adverse events for marketed products but the quality varies considerably between medical record databases, insurance claims databases, and registries of patients and prescriptions. There are also issues of confidentiality and a lack of information on 'channelling bias' i.e. the criteria that influence the selection of particular treatments for (or by) different patients. Spontaneous reporting of adverse events is notoriously incomplete and reporting rates change with time over the product's lifecycle, with a drop-off in reporting rates after 10 years. Head-to-head trials may be advocated as the 'gold standard' for obtaining comparative post-marketing data but these are extremely expensive and often very lengthy. Meta-analyses often use non-adjudicated endpoints, which confound results (e.g. Avandia and myocardial infarcts).

The 'hierarchy' of data quality needs to be taken into account and integrated into a benefit–risk assessment: Data from spontaneous reporting and epidemiological studies have less credibility than the results of RCTs, but need to be addressed, especially during the post-approval period. Patient and physician preferences are not currently captured other than through ad hoc assessments by patient representatives at expert committees or through small panels of expert physicians. A mechanism is needed for a more systematic collection of data on preferences and perceived problems and therapeutic benefits.

Options for taking post-approval benefit–risk assessment forward

The workshop (2008) considered the formation of a benefit–risk forum with regulatory authorities, pharmaceutical companies patient/public and clinician membership to be essential in order to provide a seamless link among the stakeholders as well as fostering an environment where it was believed the following issues could be debated.

- Good practices. The development of standardized procedures or good analysis practices for post-approval benefit–risk assessment.

- Off-label usage. A separate analysis might be carried out for the benefits and risks associated with off-label use.

- Comparison with older drugs whose safety profile may not be well characterized may require new data generation on the comparator in the post-approval situation.

- Concomitant medication might need to be included as a variable in the benefit–risk profile and methods for dealing with this will need to be developed.

- New biological entities (NBEs) typically require longer-term follow-up than other products and may be dependent on data from registries. For example, for vaccines, the Vaccine Safety Datalink has been an excellent database for assessing benefits and risks in disease reduction through immunisation. There is currently no similar resource for drugs but FDA's Sentinel Initiative (on medical product safety) and the European Network of Epidemiology are working in similar areas.

- Possible case studies. The forum could look at specific cases where there have been discrepant decisions on marketing approval by, for example, FDA and EMEA and/or cases where other, smaller agencies have reached different conclusions from the lead agencies. For example, Tysabri (natalizumab) is authorised for multiple sclerosis by FDA and EMEA but an extension to Crohn's disease was accepted by FDA but refused by the CHMP.

Other elements of importance for consideration in benefit–risk assessment

Value of secondary endpoints

There are different views with regard to the use of secondary endpoints in benefit–risk assessment. The regulatory review normally focuses on the primary use of the product in the target labelling, but secondary outcomes, especially where these have quality-of-life benefits, might have much greater weight if the benefit–risk assessment is made from the patient perspective. Therefore, both secondary endpoints and non-pivotal trials should be accommodated within the framework.

Patient compliance

The item in the benefit–risk framework relating to 'patient compliance' requires clarification. This could be interpreted in different ways: as a measure of patients 'lost to follow up' as they fail to complete the trials or as a projected measure of whether patients will take the medicine, once authorized, in accordance with the labelled instructions.

Best practices

Since actual practice of benefit–risk assessments is at a relatively early stage, in addition to the 'building blocks' of the framework (data definitions, ranges of 'acceptability', a priori specifications etc) consideration might be given to drawing up 'Guiding principles'.

End of phase II

It is essential to see whether the proposed framework is applicable to the decision-making process at the end-of-phase II or proof of concept stage. The objective would be to define the boundaries of acceptable safety and help inform the patient exposure required in Phase III. Whilst standards are set for demonstrating efficacy, there are no parallel guidelines for determining acceptable safety, in relation to efficacy. It might be possible, for a given effect size, to specify the acceptable risk level and hence calculate a realistic trial size. Patients would accept a higher possibility of risk for a product with major symptomatic or therapeutic benefits, when the condition is serious and/or debilitating.

A future benefit–risk framework

Based on the material presented in this chapter and the outcome of the Institute workshop in 2008, a working benefit–risk framework is proposed. The construction of the framework presented in Tables 6.5, 6.6 and 6.7 was the consensus of the workshop participants. It is noted that where an item should be considered 'high priority, and where opinions were divided, the item was accepted for routine inclusion in the framework, but designated as 'important'. Some parameters were felt to be relevant only on a case-by-case basis and not as a routine requirement.

Table 6.5 A future benefit–risk framework – safety parameters[a]

Parameter	Notes
Overall incidence of serious adverse effects	High priority for inclusion
Discontinuation rate due to adverse effects	High priority for inclusion but discontinuation due to other parameters, e.g. lack of efficacy also needs to be taken into account
Incidence, seriousness and duration of specific adverse effects, also characterised according to reversibility, latency, preventability and manageability. Adverse effects recorded from trials and marketed use, under labelled conditions	High priority for inclusion
Extrapolation of the safety profile to the target population for the labelled indication (e.g. long-term safety, potential for rare adverse effects and steepness of the dose–response curve)	High priority for inclusion; The size of the safety population, potential risks and long-term safety for chronic use products are important to consider
Adverse effects of the pharmacological class and of other classes for this indication	High priority for inclusion
Safety in subgroups, e.g. age, race, sex, polymorphic metabolism, patients with renal insufficiency, patients with hepatic insufficiency	Important for inclusion even if data is only available on a case-by-case basis
Issues raised by non-clinical data	Important for inclusion but with the caveat that animal model findings may not be predictive or relevant
Overall incidence of adverse effects (broken down into categories)	Not a high priority for all products but appropriate on a case-by-case basis; Less important than serious and specific adverse events
Demonstrated interactions with other drugs and with food	Not a high priority for all products but appropriate on a case-by-case basis in the context of the significance of the interaction for the target patient population
Potential safety risks with off-label use (including overdose)	Not a high priority for all products but appropriate on a case-by-case basis when there is a specific likelihood of off-label use; This may be a life cycle rather than a registration issue
Safety elements that can be prevented by specific measures e.g. screening, risk evaluation and mitigation strategies (REMS), vaccination, pregnancy testing etc.	Addition to the original list; Appropriate on a case-by-case basis
Transmission of adverse effectss to close contacts in the case of vaccines and immunologicals	Addition to the original list; Appropriate on a case-by-case basis

CMR Institute report, 2008.

[a] A draft schedule has been produced of parameters that could be taken into consideration in trying to formulate a benefit–risk framework, which would be applicable across different companies and different regulatory bodies. Parameters have been 'ranked' according to whether they are essential for all benefit–risk assessments, important on a case-by-case basis or of little relevance to the framework.

Table 6.6   A future benefit–risk framework – efficacy parameters

Parameter	Notes
Magnitude of the treatment effect as obtained from the results of the (primary) endpoint(s) of the pivotal clinical trials	High priority for inclusion
Clinical relevance of the magnitude of the treatment effect	High priority for inclusion (but it should relate to the threshold effect)
Statistical significance (*p*-values, confidence intervals) for the treatment effect	High priority for inclusion (*Exceptions*: No *p*-values for adaptive trials with Bayesian stats or bioterrorism products)
Relevance of the (primary) endpoint(s) of the pivotal clinical trials	High priority for inclusion
Relevance of the studied population of the pivotal clinical trials	High priority for inclusion
Discussions on dose (e.g. dose–response, minimally effective dose, etc.)	High priority for inclusion
Methodology issues beyond statistical *p*-values, e.g. multiplicity issues and *post-hoc* analyses	Essential for inclusion but could be included as a parameters in trial design and not as a separate point
Statistical/design robustness of the pivotal clinical trials (e.g. absence of bias, results replicated in second trial)	Important for inclusion but may perhaps be incorporated in an uncertainty measure
Discussions on the comparator	Important for inclusion but must be distinct from the parameter on trial design (above)
Validation of scales and outcome measures	Important for inclusion but could be a separate item or included in other parameters (e.g. patient outcomes); Validation of biomarkers is important
Evidence for the efficacy in relevant subgroups in the pivotal clinical trials according to baseline characteristics	Not a high priority for all products but appropriate on a case-by-case basis
Confirmation of treatment effect by results of secondary endpoints and the results of non-pivotal trials	Not a high priority for all products but appropriate on a case-by-case basis, especially where the secondary endpoint gives a major patient benefit; This can be split (secondary endpoints and non-pivotal results)
Patient reported outcomes whenever available	Not a high priority at registration but would have a role in life-cycle benefit–risk assessment
Anticipated compliance of patients	Borderline importance; this is possibly due to different interpretations of 'compliance' (adherence to the trial protocol or adherence to the approved labelling)

Patient convenience of dosage form	Addition to the original list: appropriate on a case-by case basis
Special conditions of use (pandemic, terrorist attack)	Addition to the original list: appropriate on a case-by-case basis
Maintenance of effect for some diseases e.g. schizophrenia, depression	Addition to the original list: appropriate on a case-by-case basis

CMR Institute report, 2008.

Table 6.7 A future benefit–risk framework – constructing benefit–risk balance

Parameter	Notes
Description of the alternative therapies or interventions (where relevant), i.e. clear description of the medical need	High priority for inclusion
Calculation of the uncertainties on benefit and risk, i.e. the amount and precision of available data	High priority for inclusion
Direct comparison (within product) of the absolute gains (efficacy) versus harms (safety) in terms of lives saved or lost, or in terms of specific clinical events	High priority for inclusion
Evaluation of the level of risk that would be acceptable with regards to the level of clinical benefit in the specific context	High priority for inclusion; Must take account of existing products and also whether an acceptable level of risk relates to a patient or a regulatory perspective
Evolution of the benefit–risk balance over time and its sensitivity to various assumptions. To be assessed: as observations increase; as the prescribed population changes; as the environment changes	High priority for inclusion
Evaluation of a benefit–risk balance in each major patient subpopulation, including pharmacogenomic subgroups	Not a high priority for all products but appropriate on a case-by-case basis; Studies may not be powered to achieve this evaluation at registration but might be applicable in life cycle management
Identification of any outstanding issues and potential post-marketing commitments in this regard	Not a priority; Not necessary if potential risks are in the model; Should be an offshoot of earlier parameters
Consideration of the different regulatory options for approval (e.g. standard marketing authorization, conditional/ priority marketing authorization)	Not a priority; this relates more to the outcome of the model

CMR International Institute for Regulatory Science Workshop, 2008.

6.6 CONCLUSION

Arguments have been developed in this book leading to the proposed MCDA approach to developing a model for the benefit–risk assessment of medicines which should be considered as one possible way forward. However, for this to be implemented as a working model (described in Chapter 5), it needs to be further developed and validated to determine for which situations it is applicable and whether it is feasible and practical to be used by pharmaceutical companies during drug development and by regulatory authorities in the review of medicines.

The barriers and solutions to developing such a model have been reviewed together with a number of issues that must be considered in developing a framework for the benefit–risk appraisal of medicines. While a quantitative approach was presented in Chapter 5, the consensus at the CMR Workshop reviewed in this chapter was that a qualitative or semiqualitative framework might be a better alternative or at least a starting point to the adoption of a more systematic approach to decision-making.

For this to be considered seriously, the first step, as previously described, is to identify the safety parameters and efficacy parameters and to address the key issues in the construction of a benefit–risk framework (Tables 6.5–6.7). However, the list is extensive and what ultimately needs to be included has to be considered on a case-by-case basis. The benefit and risk parameters to be included in the overall assessment should be put into a value tree as reviewed in Chapter 5.

The next stage required within this framework is to make a subjective assessment of the value for each parameter with respect to the therapeutic options considered in the development of this value tree. The determination of benefits and uncertainties as well as risks and uncertainties should then be reviewed and the principle of putting a value on these parameters and also a weighting is considered critical to adequately describing and producing a paper trail for this decision-making process.

The determination of the benefit–risk balance or profile is the final step in order to conclude as to whether the benefit–risk balance is positive with respect to the specified product and indication.

To date, this approach in qualitative terms is described above and is being addressed by a number of groups as indicated in the appendices. The importance of developing a framework for benefit–risk assessment of medicines is critical and further work over the next few years including all relevant stakeholders, will hopefully enable this research methodology, improve the development of medicines and inform regulatory authorities and practicing physicians as to how to make this decision-making process more robust and transparent. This will ensure an improved approach to making more appropriate benefit–risk assessments which could result in safer, more effective medicines reaching the market.

Beyond complexity lies simplicity
('as simple as possible and no simpler' – Albert Einstein)

Summary Reports of the CMR International Institute for Regulatory Science March 2004 and June 2005 Workshops on Benefit–Risk

Summary Report of the Workshop on The Development of a Model for Benefit–risk Assessment of Medicines Based on Multi-Criteria Decision Analysis organized by the CMR International Institute for Regulatory Science and Cardiff University

SUMMARY REPORT

A1.1 OVERVIEW

Determining the benefit–risk balance of a medicine is one of the most important steps in its development, review and post-approval re-assessment but there are currently no well-established, validated models for this essential task. The objective of this interactive Workshop convened by the CMR International Institute for Regulatory Science was to examine a proposal for the development of a new model for benefit–risk assessment using Multi-Criteria Decision Analysis (MCDA). This is a method of

Benefit-Risk Appraisal of Medicines   Filip Mussen, Sam Salek, Stuart Walker
© 2009 John Wiley & Sons, Ltd

looking at complex problems, of breaking the problem into more manageable pieces in order to allow data and judgements to be brought to bear on different aspect, and then of reassembling the pieces to present a coherent overall picture for decision makers. The purpose of this tool is to serve as an aid to thinking and decision making, but not to take the decision.

The Institute Workshop brought together senior experts from regulatory agencies and the pharmaceutical industry involved in the development, assessment and post-approval safety assessment of medicines for a preliminary evaluation of the model (see participants list). The one-and-a-half day meeting was conducted as an interactive working session with the assistance of a facilitator, Professor Larry Philips, an expert in the techniques of 'Decision Conferencing' as well as MCDA. The proposed benefit–risk model was discussed and tested using a case study based on actual, but anonymized data.

Although time allowed only a relatively simple example to be discussed, participants were unanimous in agreeing that the methodology had great potential for addressing benefit–risk assessments and there was a strong wish to carry the project forward. From the industry point of view it was perceived as a means not only to enhance in-house decision-making processes about the viability of R&D projects but also to anticipate potential problems before an application is submitted for agency review. The regulators were keen to test the model further using retrospective and prospective data with a view to gauging its value in improving the consistency and transparency of the decision-making process.

It was strongly recommended that the CMR International Institute should follow up this initiative with further Workshops, as soon as possible. In the meantime both regulatory and industry participants expressed the wish to study the technique further and learn more about the MCDA methodology.

A1.2   FORMAT OF THE WORKSHOP

The main focus of the meeting was the live, interactive demonstration of the MCDA model, using the case study, in which delegates participated in the role of the assessors and the model was developed and tested 'on screen' using customized Hiview software. Before starting work on the case study Filip Mussen (Research Fellow developing the model as part of his doctoral thesis) presented an overview of the criteria and current methods for benefit–risk analysis (Annex 1) and Professor Larry Philips introduced the principles of MCDA. There was a wide ranging discussion on the concepts of the benefits of a medicine, in terms of efficacy, effectiveness and implications for the individual and public health as well as the assessment of risk and the differences in risk perception between the scientific and regulatory community and the public (see Annex 2).

A1.3   THE MCDA MODEL

The model discussed by the group and developed from the case study is presented here in broad outline only. The case study related to a hypothetical new recombinant tumour necrosis factor-α (TNF-α) receptor inhibitor indicated for the treatment of active rheumatoid arthritis resistant to other treatments, including methotrexate. Data on outcomes and adverse event reports were given for clinical trials on the drug alone against placebo and on the drug with concomitant use of methotrexate.

The first step in the MCDA model is to identify the *Options* for the possible outcome of the benefit–risk assessment. There might normally be only two options: that benefits outweigh risks (the product is the 'option' for treatment) or that risks outweigh benefits (the comparator or placebo is the option). In the specific case study, however, three outcome options were identified: the product, the product plus methotrexate and the placebo.

The second step is to identify the *Criteria* to be taken into account in determining the outcome ('option') for the assessment and to group these criteria under the two main headings of 'benefit' and 'risk'. In the case study, the criteria for benefit included results of the clinical studies measured as the percentage of patients achieving specific endpoints for symptomatic relief and slowing of disease progression. The criteria for risk included not only the incidence of adverse events and drug-related reactions, but also unobserved but potential risks based on knowledge of factors including related products, mechanism of action and likelihood of immunosuppression.

The software converts the criteria into a diagram described as the 'value tree' which gives a hierarchical structure for the factors contributing to the benefit–risk balance. In a series of steps, assisted by the computer software, each criteria is assigned a *Score* and each score is given a *Weight* according to its relative importance to the benefit–risk decision. Weighted scores are calculated at each level in the hierarchy which enables an overall weighted score to be calculated for each of the options.

The process of 'scoring' is based predominantly on measurable data such as the clinical trial endpoints and incidence of adverse events, measured as percentages. Other scores, for example the risk of potential but unobserved reactions must, of necessity, be more subjective but the methodology, nonetheless, allows a numerical 'score' assigned to such imprecise criteria.

The process of 'weighting' the scores is where experience and judgement are built into the methodology. The assignment of weight to a score is normally based on a combination of factors on which a value judgement is made, for example the scale of difference between the results for a drug and placebo in achieving symptomatic relief and the relative importance of demonstrating symptomatic relief over showing that the disease process has slowed.

A1.4   SENSITIVITY TESTING AND RESULTS

The 'subjective' element of scoring and weighting raised some concerns among participants, although it was accepted that, by their very nature, determinations of benefit–risk could never be based solely on objective evaluations of hard data. An important feature of the MCDA model and software, however, is the ability to carry out sensitivity analyses on the results by varying any of the weights and scores to assess the impact on the overall benefit–risk balance. Sensitivity analyses were demonstrated for some of the scoring and weighting decisions from the case study, where there had been differences of opinion amongst those present. Participants were surprised to note that, in several cases where the differences had appeared major, the impact on the overall outcome was scarcely significant.

The outcome for the particular case study and MCDA model tested at the Workshop was that the option with the optimal benefit-to-risk balance was the drug with concomitant methotrexate treatment. Participants were impressed to be informed that this was the 'real life' outcome for the assessment of the TNF-α receptor inhibitor, Remicade (inflixmab).

A1.5   WHAT WAS GAINED FROM THE WORKSHOP

Participants agreed that the workshop had been an important initial step towards developing a model with significant potential benefits for both companies and regulators. Multi-Criteria Decision Analysis, techniques in combination with the software, provide possibilities for a dynamic model that can be developed and modified to meet a variety of scenarios encountered in drug development and evaluation.

The advantages of the MCDA technique that were identified during the meeting, included possibilities for:

- enhancing the consistency and objectivity and transparency of the decision-making process for benefit–risk assessments by providing a structured and systematic approach and a 'paper trail' for tracking the process and providing greater accountability

- reviewing the consistency of regulatory decisions on marketing authorization applications (MAA) in order to learn from past experience

- achieving a better understanding and more rational explanations of why different agencies reach different conclusions on the basis of the same data

- providing a training tool for both agency and industry staff involved in the development and assessment of new products

- allowing industry to test the benefit–risk data for new products before submitting an application, in order to identify areas where data may need to be strengthened or clarified

- carrying out more balanced and objective benefit–risk re-assessments in post-authorization situations where there is a tendency to focus primarily on adverse event reporting.

A1.6   THE NEXT STEPS

Participants urged the CMR International Institute to convene other interactive workshops using 'decision conferencing' techniques to explore further the possibilities of the MCDA methodology.

Acknowledging that the participation at this Workshop was predominantly European, Professor Walker proposed that priority should be given to a meeting in the USA in order to see if similar results and acceptance of the model would be achieved with FDA participation and more US company experts.

It was also suggested that more time should be allowed for subsequent workshops so that there could be industry and regulatory break-out sessions in order to see how different viewpoints impact on the scoring and weighting for benefit and risk.

Both industry and agency participants were keen to ensure that the impetus was not lost, in the meantime and wished to test the model further within their own environment.

Following the meeting possibilities for taking the project further in the EU were discussed with the EMEA.

It is proposed that the CMR International Institute for Regulatory Science should act as the primary contact point for companies and regulatory agencies that wish to follow-up this project and receive further information and contacts for developing the use of the MCDA model for benefit risk assessment.

A1.7   ACKNOWLEDGEMENTS

1 Multi-criteria decision analysis was implemented in this project with the use of Hiview software, which was developed at the London School of Economics and is marketed by Catalyze Limited. Further information can be obtained at www.catalyze.co.uk.

Due to confidentiality reasons only a summary of this workshop is provided in this book; however the full report can be provided to those interested on application to CMR International Institute for Regulatory Science.

Workshop participants

Facilitator

Professor Larry Phillips	Professor of Decision Analysis, London School of Economics

Delegates

Professor Gunnar Alván	Director General, Medical Products Agency, Sweden
Dr Daniel Brasseur	Chairman, Committee for Proprietary Medicinal Products (CPMP), EMEA
Dr Graham Burton	Senior Vice President, Celgene Corporation, USA
Dr. Janice Bush	Vice President, Safety Strategy and Liaison, Johnson & Johnson, USA
Ms Margaret Cone	Director of Regulatory Science, CMR International Institute for Regulatory Science
Dr Moira Daniels	Director, Global Regulatory Information and Intelligence, AstraZeneca Pharmaceuticals, UK
Dr Bryan Garber	Health Risk Management, Health Canada
Dr. Paul Huckle	Senior Vice President, GlaxoSmithKline R&D, UK.
Dr. David Jefferys	Head of Devices Sector, Medicines and Health Products, Regulatory Agency (MHRA), UK.
Dr. Patrick Le Courtois	Head of Unit for the Pre-authorisation Evaluation of Medicines for Human Use, EMEA
Dr Neil McAuslane	Chief Scientific Officer, CMR International Ltd
Mr. Filip Mussen	Director, Regulatory Affairs Europe, Merck Research Laboratories, Belgium
Dr. Sam Salek	Senior Lecturer, Department of Clinical Pharmacology, University of Wales, Cardiff
Dr. Tomas P Salmonson	CPMP Representative, Medical Products Agency, Sweden.
Dr. Valerie Simmons	Advisor, Global Product Safety, Lilly Research Laboratories, U.K.
Professor Stuart Walker	President and Founder, CMR International Limited, U.K.
Dr Beat Von Graffenreid	Division of Biotechnology Medicines, Swissmedic, Switzerland

ANNEX 1

A1.8   OVERVIEW OF THE CRITERIA AND CURRENT METHODS FOR BENEFIT–RISK ANALYSIS:

Definitions in benefit–risk assessment

- *Benefit*: the proven therapeutic good of a product; should also include the patient's subjective assessment of its effects (WHO Collaborating Centre).

- *Risk*: the probability of harm being caused; the probability (chance, odds) of an occurrence (WHO Collaborating Centre).

- *Benefit* and risk are evaluative terms which contain value judgements (clinical studies cannot determine whether an effect is a benefit/risk, and how beneficial/ harmful the effect is).

- *Benefit–risk balance*: more accurate than benefit–risk ratio (benefits and risks are not of the same nature).

Five concepts in benefit–risk assessment

- A separate benefit–risk balance for each indication.

- All available data should be considered in benefit–risk assessment.

- The nature of the disease should be taken into account for benefit–risk balance.

- Absolute versus relative benefit–risk balance (compare with alternative therapies?).

- The benefit–risk balance is dynamic and evolves over time.

Criteria to consider in benefit–risk assessment

The criteria selected are based on EU, FDA and ICH guidance. (The numbers in brackets refer to the 20 responses – 14 companies, 6 agencies – to questions in a CMR survey in 2002 that asked which factors should be included in a model for benefit risk assessment)

Benefit

For each pivotal trial:

- efficacy (primary endpoint) versus comparator and its clinical relevance *(20/20)*
- statistical significance of the efficacy results *(18/20)*
- clinical relevance of the primary endpoints *(19/20)*
- representivity of the studied population for the population targeted in the label *(18/20)*
- evidence for the efficacy in relevant subgroups *(14/20)*
- design, conduct and statistical adequacy of the trial *(18/20)*
- confirmation of treatment effect by results of non-primary endpoints *(16/20)*.

General benefit criteria:

- confirmation of efficacy by results of relevant non-pivotal trials and extensions *(16/20)*

- anticipated patient compliance *(11/20)*

- clustering (consistency) of results of the pivotal trials.

Risk

- Overall incidence of adverse effects (from clinical trials) *(16/20)*.

- Overall incidence of serious adverse effects (from clinical trials) *(20/20)*.

- Discontinuation rate due to adverse effects (from clinical trials) *(15/20)*.

- Incidence, seriousness and duration of specific adverse effects (from clinical trials and post-marketing surveillance) *(20/20)*.

- Interactions with other drugs and with food *(18/20)*.

- Safety in subgroups (e.g. age, race, sex) *(20/20)*.

- Potential for off-label use leading to safety hazards *(12/20)*.

- Potential for non-demonstrated additional risk due to limitations of clinical trials and/or short market exposure.

- Potential for non-demonstrated additional risk due to safety issues observed in preclinical safety studies but not in humans.

- Potential for non-demonstrated additional risk due to safety issues observed with other medicines of the same pharmacological class.

(The latter three criteria were previously clustered in the survey as 'generalizability of the safety profile to the general population' (18/20).)

A1.9   WHY WOULD MODELS FOR BENEFIT–RISK ASSESSMENT BE USEFUL?

- Enhance consistency in expressing the benefit–risk balance of a product.

- Enhance objectivity in recommendations/ decisions on the benefit–risk of a product (by Registration Committees and in Marketing Authorization Applications).

- Increase transparency of regulatory decisions (approval and post-approval).

- Force the assessor to focus on benefits and risks.

- Ideally, could be used as a tool to compare products.

- Can be used as a tool for regulators and industry, but cannot substitute for the final decision-making.

A1.10   OBJECTIVES FOR A NEW MODEL

A model which:

- is able to take into account the data in the MAA or otherwise available to regulatory agencies (i.e. safety and efficacy data from multiple clinical trials, post-approval AE data); no cost-benefit data

- requires no additional analyses of source data (safety and efficacy), or meta-analyses

- closely matches the current regulatory agency practices for benefit–risk assessment

- can be used during initial registration and post-approval

- can be validated

- is applicable to all kind of drugs, including vaccines and OTC drugs.

Which models are currently available?

Currently there are no well-established, validated models (qualitative or quantitative) although a few models are described in the literature:

- 'Principle of threes' (Edwards *et al.*, 1996)

- TURBO model (Amery, 1998)

- Evidence-based benefit and risk concept (Beckmann, 1999).

These three models were mainly developed for pharmacovigilance purposes: post-marketing re-assessment (the 'Principles of Threes' model and the TURBO model are described in the CIOMS IV report).

Other models have been developed to assess the benefit–risk based on one clinical trial, for example:

- 'Benefit-Less-Risk Analysis' (Chuang-Stein)

- Mathematical model based on Numbers Needed to Treat (NNT) & Numbers Needed to Harm (NNH) (Schulzer & Mancini)

- 'Principle of threes' grading system (Edwards *et al.*).

A1.11   WEAKNESSES OF THE CURRENT MODELS

- Many criteria in the models are not well defined with regard to the type, quality and relative importance of the data to be taken into account.

- Models do not take into account many of the benefit and risk criteria previously identified.

- Models are not very sophisticated and allow only a very crude benefit–risk assessment.

- Models have not been validated nor broadly used in practice.

ANNEX 2

A1.12   POINTS FROM THE WORKSHOP DISCUSSIONS

Historical perspective

Professor Stuart Walker provided an overview of the historical and present role of CMR International Institute for Regulatory Science bringing together senior experts from the pharmaceutical industry and international regulatory agencies to address issues of policy and practice that impact on the development and evaluation of new medicines.[1] He noted that CMR had first addressed Risk Benefit assessment at a Workshop in 1985. Professor Walker emphasized the extent to which the subject has moved on by remarking that industry, at that time, was very resistant to economic issues being raised in relation to the assessment of medicines and somewhat dismissive of the concept that 'quality of life' could be a measurable factor in assessing the benefit of medicines.

In one important respect, however, benefit–risk assessment has not moved on. The re-evaluation of benefit–risk after authorization is predominantly focused on risk – reports of adverse events and misuse – and the benefit of a medicine is rarely reviewed with a consequence that the benefit–risk almost inevitably appears worse with passing time.

Need for a benefit–risk model

The general discussions of the need for a viable benefit–risk model included the following points:

- the need for a better understanding of why different agencies come to different conclusions when faced with essentially the same application data

- the increasing pressure on agencies to increase transparency and accountability and to establish a 'paper trail' to explain how decisions are reached

- the need for a system that is sufficiently dynamic and flexible that it can be developed with experience with the potential that its application could be extended to include the views of a wider range of stakeholders, including patients and physicians

- acknowledgement that current approaches are somewhat haphazard not only on the part of the regulators, where decisions can be inconsistent but also on the part of companies where data in submissions on benefits and risks is not presented in a coherent and well structured manner.

Benefit goes beyond efficacy

It was agreed that discussions of the benefits of a medicine must encompass more than the measurement of efficacy in the clinical setting. Other factors include the following.

- Social settings and how the disease is managed in society, for example the added value of being able to treat a patient at home.

- The relative merits of a small improvement in a large number of individuals versus a major improvement that is only seen in some individuals.

- The different perception of improvement that a patient and doctor may have. For example a relatively small clinical improvement in mobility may represent a major lifestyle change for the individual patient. Conversely clinicians might see great value in a drug that halts disease progress but this is of little benefit to the patient if the symptoms of the disease are not relieved.

There was also a discussion of the need to distinguish between the *efficacy* of a medicine, as evaluated in clinical trials and the *effectiveness* of a medicine that can only be judged once it has found its place in the clinical practice, post-authorization.

Role of value judgements

It was acknowledged that value judgement is an integral part of benefit–risk assessment. Although it may be possible to draw up guidelines for the minimum data set that must be submitted to support a benefit–risk assessment, the decision making process will always include the application of informed opinion that is outside the scope of the data on its own. This is in contrast to the need to prove efficacy alone, which is often written into legal requirements. The MCDA model incorporates value judgement into the system of 'weighting' the values placed on different criteria used in the assessment.

Experts may disagree

History and experience has shown that there is no single 'correct' opinion on a matter as subjective as benefit–risk evaluation and there will always be disagreement among experts. Part of the purpose of introducing a model for assessing benefit–risk, however, is to move away from the scenario of discussions behind closed doors from which decisions emerge from 'smoke filled rooms' without explanations or accountability. A model that is applied transparently and consistently would also diminish the all-too-common scenario where a decision, apparently made by a committee of peers, is unduly influenced by vociferous and dominant individuals.

Perception of risk

Assessment of risk cannot be based on scientific and statistical factors alone. The 'perception' of risk, especially by the public is extremely subjective and has been studied extensively. There was a discussion, at the workshop, of the concept that public perception of risk is based on three factors: *dread* (e.g. bovine spongiform encephalopathy transmission to humans), *unknown* (e.g. effects of mumps, measles and rubella vaccination, MMR) and *numbers* involved (e.g. motor accidents).[1] Results of studies based on these factors show that, against all statistical arguments, the risks of human variant Creutztfeld–Jakob disease are perceived as a much more serious than, for example, road accidents.

It was emphasized that training about making judgements on risk must include training on the nature of risk perception.

Models for efficacy

It was noted that, whilst there are regulatory guidelines on the data required to support claims for efficacy, there is no 'model' for assessing whether efficacy has been demonstrated. In particular, there appears little discussion on the number of patients that show improvement when treated vs the magnitude and nature of that improvement which could range from:

- symptomatic relief;
- slowing of disease progression; to
- curing the disease.

Role of comparators

Notwithstanding moves to harmonize the use of comparators in clinical trials, there remains a significant difference in practices between the United States, where proof of efficacy against inactive placebo is accepted and Europe, where active comparators are expected in trials to prove efficacy and 'non-inferiority'.

There was a discussion of the issues involved when a new medicine is the first in its class and the implications for evaluating benefit and risk against active comparators with a significantly different mode of action. The question was also raised of whether judgements on the benefit of a first-in-class medicine are influenced by knowledge that similar drugs are in the pipeline.

Does the nature of disease impact judgements on benefits?

There was discussion on whether the seriousness of the disease is automatically a factor in assessing benefit. There is a tendency to regard drugs that benefit patients with a life-threatening disease, even when the improvement is only symptomatic, as having a greater value than a medicine for the treatment of a less severe or self-limiting condition. The example discussed was an anti-nauseant used for cancer patients undergoing chemotherapy and one recommended for sea-sickness.

Sequential decisions

Historically, as noted earlier, monitoring the way benefit–risk changes with time has focussed on risk and cumulative reports of adverse events and side effects. The benefit–risk assessment model should ensure that information on benefit is taken into consideration in a more balanced way when it becomes necessary to re-assess the safety of a product. An important factor is the increased trend towards 'conditional' approvals with commitments to carry out post-approval studies, requiring subsequent evaluation for any impact on the benefit–risk balance.

Effects of how regulators perceive their role

Not only do experts within one regulatory system disagree, but different conclusions are often reached between regulatory agencies. This can be, in part, the result of differing views of the role of regulation and the balance between responsibility to the individual patient and the population as a whole. Other factors may include:

- the impact and influence of the views of stakeholders including patients associations, physicians, health activists and reimbursement agencies

- the application of the 'precautionary principle' resulting in very low risk tolerance

- political influences placed agencies when dealing with high-profile diseases (e.g. AIDS) and emotive issues where there is a degree of 'unknowns (e.g. MMR vaccine).

Communication of risk

Some medicines have known, serious adverse consequences for specific groups of patients (e.g. the elderly) or in pre-existing conditions. If the benefits, for eligible patients, are significant, can the 'risk' side of the equation be reduced by appropriate cautions and warnings in the product information (labeling)? There was general agreement that labeling and proposals for risk management and communication should be included in the model. It was also acknowledged, however, that experience has shown how difficult it is to ensure that physicians heed the warnings in product information.

Potential for off-label use

It follows, from the previous point, that the potential for off-label use must be a factor in deciding on the weighting to be assigned to specific and 'class' risks associated with a product. Off label use may not only relate to ignored warnings and contraindications, however. It may take the form of using the product in extended, related indications, that are not explicitly included in the labeling. This may, in the long run, reveal new 'benefits' of the medicine.

Benefit–risk Assessment Model for Medicines: Developing a Structured Approach to Decision Making

Report of the Workshop organized by the CMR International Institute for Regulatory Science and Cardiff University at the Georgetown Inn, Washington DC, USA, 13–14 June 2005

SUMMARY REPORT

A1.13   OVERVIEW

As public accountability grows for decisions taken in both public and private sectors, so the need develops for organizations to provide an audit trail for important decisions. Decisions leading to drug approvals demand careful attention with respect to balancing the benefits and risks, which in turn requires a structured process that leaves an audit trail.

The Workshop brought together twenty-seven senior participants drawn from regulatory agencies in the United States and Europe, academia and the pharmaceutical industry (see Annex 1). The purpose was to explore a structured model for benefit–risk assessment and consider its potential for providing support to decision-makers in both regulatory agencies and pharmaceutical companies.

This was the second Workshop on this topic, hosted by the CMR International Institute for Regulatory Science, the first having been held in March 2004, in the UK. The success of this meeting led recommendations for a further Workshop to be convened in the United States.

The Workshop was organized to encourage frank and open discussions about the way in which important, far-reaching decisions are taken within both companies and regulatory agencies and the potential shortcomings of such processes. The main component of the meeting, however, was an interactive demonstration of the application of the technical model 'multi-criteria decision analysis' (MCDA). The model was discussed using a hypothetical scenario based on safety and efficacy data relating to an atypical antipsychotic agent that was clinically tested against placebo and a comparator compound.

The MCDA methodology provides a way of looking at complex problems and breaking them down into more manageable pieces that can be studied using a mixture of data and judgement. The components are then 're-assembled', using computer software, to present a coherent overall picture for the decision makers. The purpose of this tool is to serve as an aid to thinking and decision-making, but not to take the decisions.

At the conclusion of the meeting it was, as at the 2004 meeting, unanimously agreed that the methodology had great potential and it was recommended that it should be explored further as an adjunct to the decision-making process for both companies and regulatory agencies. An important part of this would be to undertake retrospective testing using actual case studies.

It was also recommended that a third Workshop should be convened at a later stage to discuss the results of such studies and explore further the practical application of the methodology and its place in preparing regulatory submissions as well as in the regulatory review process.

Background

The CMR International institute for Regulatory Science became actively involved in the application of MCDA methodology to the benefit–risk assessment of medicines through the research project undertaken by Dr Filip Mussen, MSD Europe, as part of his doctoral thesis, when studying for a PhD as an Institute Scholar[1].

The previous Workshop held in March 2004 was convened at the London School of Economics when the MCDA model was demonstrated using a case study based on a novel treatment for active rheumatoid arthritis. As background to the discussions a summary of criteria and current methods for benefit–risk analysis was presented by Filip Mussen and this is given in Annex 2 to this report.

Participants at the first Workshop were enthusiastic about the MCDA methodology but it was acknowledged that participation had been predominantly European and one of the recommendations was to hold a similar meeting in the United States in order to capture the North American perspective, and with the active participation of the FDA.

---

[1] PhD thesis entitled 'The evaluation of methods for benefit-risk assessment of medicines and the development of a new model using multi-criteria decision analysis'. Studies undertaken at the University of Wales, Cardiff, under the supervision of Professor Sam Selek, Welsh School of Pharmacy, and Professor Stuart Walker, CMR International

Format and style of the workshop

The second Workshop started from the premise, agreed at the London meeting, that decisions on benefit–risk that decide the fate of a new medicine must be made in a consistent and transparent manner that weighs up the evidence of efficacy and safety objectively, whilst allowing judgement to be exercised.

In the introductory session, participants were asked to outline their experiences and concerns that made them interested in participating in the Workshop. An important driver was the fact that an increasing number of individuals within both companies and agencies are becoming involved in decision-making processes, at all management levels, and there were concerns about the lack of structure and guidance on such processes.

In industry, assessment of the benefit and risks is a continuous process throughout R&D and extends into risk management strategies for products once they are authorized. Management decisions on whether to terminate the development of a new product must take account of commercial risks as well as scientific views on the safety of the product.

The benefit–risk assessments made by regulators may have more clearly defined criteria for efficacy and safety, resulting from regulations and guidelines. There were, however, concerns about the need to ensure that judgement and flexibility can be exercised and that pivotal decisions are always subject to peer review.

There is also a need to take account of the concept of 'benefit' from the patients' point of view, especially in terms of quality of life. In addition, sufferers from life-threatening or chronic diseases may have a different attitude from companies and regulators when it comes to 'acceptable risk'.

A1.14   WORKSHOP CONCLUSIONS AND RECOMMENDATIONS

In the final session of the Workshop, participants were asked to reflect on the demonstration of the model and provide their observations on its application in drug development and review.

Observations

- Company members could envisage the approach being used to shape the way in which arguments on the benefit–risk balance of a new product were presented in a regulatory submission.

- FDA expressed the view that the methodology could have a valuable place in in-house decision-making by both companies and regulatory agencies but that, at present, it would not be a suitable way to present data for assessment or at a hearing.

- It was acknowledged that there might be significant organizational and 'cultural' challenges to introducing the methodology and it would require individuals with enthusiasm and conviction to overcome these.

- Consistency among agencies is a problem and the MCDA model could have a place in research into inconsistencies within agencies and differences of opinion between agencies.

- The methodology might provide greater insight into why products fail in phase III.

Recommendations

- There was a clear consensus that the participants wished to see the CMR International Institute carrying this project forward with further validation of the MCDA model.

- It was strongly recommended that CMR should undertake a specific study of the methodology, in collaboration with regulatory agencies and pharmaceutical companies, using data from 'real-world' examples from past and current cases. This might include:

- A retrospective study, including products that had failed at the pre- and post-submission stage, using the model to re-evaluate the benefit–risk decisions that had been taken;

- A pilot study, starting with early portfolio projects, in a therapeutic area such as diabetes.

- A comparison of outcomes, using the MCDA model, when applied in the United States and in the EU.

- It was agreed that the 'learning' process would benefit from a further interactive Workshop, organized on a similar basis to the current meeting, with a limited number of participants and a further 'hands-on' demonstration of the methodology.

The way forward

Project: To develop a structured approach to decision-making for benefit–risk assessment of medicines

Following the Workshop in June 2006 several immediate actions have been agreed and initiated to take this project forward:

Publications

The publication of two papers was proposed under the title '*A structured approach to the Benefit–risk Assessment of Medicines*':

1. Development of a new model using multi-criteria decision analysis (MCDA)

2. The practical application of a new model.

It has been proposed that these should be published in the journal of Clinical Pharmacoepidemiology and Drug Safety, ideally in the first half of 2006.

Further doctoral study

It was recommended that a future research programme should have the following objectives namely to:

*   identify and determine how decision-making is implemented in established drug regulatory authorities

*   identify, by means of a questionnaire, how 'best practices' are incorporated into decision-making by industry and regulatory authorities

*   refine and develop the MCDA model for benefit–risk assessment in order to optimize its practical application in real-life situations.

Incorporating the views of patients

CMR International will continue the successful formula of interactive workshops to demonstrate the model to regulatory and industry participants, as recommended by the Workshop. It is proposed that these should focus on:

*   comparing outcomes from the same scenario evaluated by different stakeholders

*   seeking ways to incorporate the views of patients, using the methodology, and evaluating the impact on outcomes.

Due to confidentiality reasons only a summary of this workshop is provided in this book; however the full report can be provided to those interested on application to CMR International Institute for Regulatory Science.

ANNEX 1

A1.15 WORKSHOP PARTICIPANTS

Dr Andre Broekmans	Vice President, Regulatory Affairs & Pharma Policy, Organon International Inc, USA
Dr George Butler	Vice President, Customer Partnerships, AstraZeneca Pharmaceuticals, USA
Dr Lyn Caltabiano	Vice President, Clinical Pharmacology Operations, GlaxoSmithKline, USA
Dr Patrizia Cavazzoni	Director, Global Drug Safety – Neuroscience, Eli Lilly & Company, USA
Dr Janine Collins	Director, Drug Safety, Celgene Europe Ltd, UK
Ms Margaret Cone	Director of Regulatory Science, CMR International Institute
Prof Bruno Flamion	Chair, Scientific Advice Working Party and CHMP Member, EMEA, UK
Dr Trevor Gibbs	Senior Vice President, Senior Physician, Medical Governance and Pharmacovigilance, GlaxoSmithKline, UK
Dr Edmund Harrigan	Senior VP, Worldwide Regulatory Affairs & Quality Assurance, Pfizer Inc, USA
Dr John Howell III	President, Portfolio Decisions Inc, USA
Dr David Jefferys	Senior Regulatory Strategic Adviser, Eisai Europe, UK
Dr John Jenkins	Director, Office of New Drugs, Center for Drug Evaluation & Research, Food and Drug Administration, USA
Dr Sandra Kweder	Deputy Director, Office of New Drugs, Center for Drug Evaluation & Research, Food and Drug Administration, USA
Prof Jan Liliemark	Scientific Director, Medical Products Agency, Sweden
Dr Murray Lumpkin	Acting Deputy Commissioner, Food and Drug Administration, USA
Dr Freeman Marvin	Principal, Innovative Decisions Inc, USA
Dr Neil McAuslane	Chief Scientific Officer, CMR International Institute
Patricia McGovern	Director, Special Projects, Novartis Pharmaceuticals Corporation, USA
Charles Monahan	Senior Regulatory Affairs Associate, Millennium Pharmaceuticals Inc, USA
Dr Filip Mussen	Associate Director, Regulatory Affairs, Merck Sharp & Dohme (Europe) Inc, Belgium
Dr Thierry Nebout	Senior Consultant, Institut de Recherches Internationales Servier, France

Professor Larry Phillips	Professor of Decision Analysis, London School of Economics, UK
Dr Atsuko Shibata	Associate Medical Director, Amgen Inc, USA
Dr Robert Temple	Associate Director for Medical Policy, Center for Drug Evaluation, Food and Drug Administration, USA
Dr Mary Ellen Turner	Vice President, Wyeth Research, USA
Prof Stuart Walker	President and Founder, CMR International
Dr Wayne Wallis	Head, Global Safety, Amgen Inc, USA

Office of Health Economics Briefing: Challenges and Opportunities for Improving Benefit–risk Assessment of Pharmaceuticals from an Economic Perspective – James Cross and Louis Garrison (August 2008)

BRIEFING NO 43 AUGUST 2008

A2.1 CHALLENGES AND OPPORTUNITIES FOR IMPROVING BENEFIT–RISK ASSESSMENT OF PHARMACEUTICALS FROM AN ECONOMIC PERSPECTIVE

James T. Cross, MS, Louis P. Garrison, PhD
University of Washington, Seattle, USA

Benefit-Risk Appraisal of Medicines Filip Mussen, Sam Salek, Stuart Walker
© 2009 John Wiley & Sons, Ltd

A2.2   EXECUTIVE SUMMARY

In October 2007, the Office of Health Economics (OHE) hosted a workshop in London on Benefit–risk Assessments for Drugs. Researchers (see Box 1) presented ideas and case studies to show how certain tools and methods used in economic analysis and the decision sciences could improve the methodology that regulatory authorities such as the European Medicines Agency (EMEA) and the US Food and Drug Administration (FDA) use to evaluate drug benefit and risk (EMEA, 2007a).

BOX A2.1 OHE WORKSHOP CONTRIBUTORS:

Eric Abadie, MD	EMBA European Medicines Agency
Andrew Briggs, MSc, DPhil	University of Glasgow
Louis Garrison, PhD	University of Washington
A. Brett Hauber, PhD	Research Triangle Institute
F. Reed Johnson, PhD	Research Triangle Institute
Larry Lynd, PhD	University of British Columbia
Lawrence Phillips, PhD	London School of Economics

Four methods were presented and discussed:

1. Health outcomes modelling using quality-adjusted life years (see Box 3)

2. Incremental Net Health Benefit (see Box 4)

3. Stated Benefit–risk Preferences (see Box 5)

4. Multi-criteria Decision Analysis (see Box 6).

The first two – representing the health impact dimension of cost-effectiveness analysis – are quite similar, comparing risks and benefits in a common metric. Health outcomes modelling can be seen as an extension or broadening of the incremental net benefit approach, which itself involves the modelling of outcomes, to include population level impacts such as the health benefits forgone in delaying an approval decision. Stated preference measurement of benefit–risk involves eliciting patient preferences among hypothetical health states. Multi-criteria decision analysis is a structured group decision-making process based on decision science.

There was agreement that each of these tools offers the potential to improve regulatory benefit–risk assessment by addressing three major issues with the current regulatory approach:

1. Transparency: To what extent are benefit–risk assessments and decisions clearly defined and justified for patients and clinicians, and others outside the regulatory process?

2. Preferences: Do or should regulators' preferences in benefit–risk trade-offs reflect those of patients or clinicians? What is the appropriate perspective that should be taken in regulatory assessments? How and should 'societal preferences' be estimated?

3. Consistency: Should the same benefit–risk assessment method be used for all therapeutic areas given differences in the quality of evidence available? No single tool has yet emerged as the clear choice to address these three issues. Yet, strong arguments were made at the OHE meeting for regulators to consider the preferences of patients and the community in some manner and each of the methods provides some scope for this paradigm. The workshop presentations and discussion highlighted the strengths and limitations of each. Further developmental work and research is needed to refine and test each of the methods and to identify the circumstances in which each would be used.

A2.3   CURRENT DRUG BENEFIT–RISK ASSESSMENT: MOTIVATION FOR INCLUDING A HEALTH ECONOMIST'S PERSPECTIVE

When a physician prescribes a drug product and a patient decides to use it, both assume that the product is generally safe and effective for its intended use-that, on average, the product's benefits (e.g. increases in life expectancy or quality-of-life) outweigh the product's risks (e.g. arrhythmia, liver failure). The EMEA's regulatory review process, first established in 1993 and since revised to its current form, specifies that the risk-benefit balance of products must be assessed for marketing authorization. (Council of the European Union 1993, 2004) Product-specific assessments are in the form of European Public Assessment Reports (EPARs) (EMEA, 2007b). An EPAR reflects the scientific conclusion of the Committee for Medicinal Products for Human Use (CHMP), summarizing the grounds for the CHMP opinion in favour of granting a marketing authorization for a specific product. The EPAR is updated throughout the authorization period as changes to the original terms and conditions of the authorization. Regulations do not specify the methods for conducting risk-benefit assessment, nor do they provide guidelines as to what constitutes a positive or negative 'risk-benefit balance.' This regulatory scenario also exists in the United States where government regulations and guidance from the FDA do not specify how data should be weighed or quantified to form an overall risk-benefit balance.

The ability of regulators adequately to assess drug benefit and risk has been repeatedly called into question. The Council for International Organizations of Medical Sciences (CIOMS) issued a report in 1998 which declared that no defined and proven method exists to evaluate benefit and risk (CIOMS, 1998). In the decade since this report, a series of increasingly publicised product withdrawals and controversial postmarketing labelling decisions has occurred, most notably the market withdrawal of rofecoxib. This ignited controversy over how new postmarketing trial data affect a product's perceived overall benefit–risk profile and methods for synthesizing various pieces of information on benefit and risk. Like the earlier CIOMS report, the recent Institute of Medicine (IOM) report on drug safety has challenged US regulators to develop novel methods of benefit–risk assessment (IOM, 2006).

Current regulatory decisions are often not transparent because they attempt to integrate the quality and quantity of a heterogeneous body of evidence presented to demonstrate efficacy and safety (FDA 1998; International Conference on Harmonisation 1998). These decisions have not explicitly weighed the relative value of each piece of evidence (such as risk estimates for different health outcomes) that inform the decision maker. The regulatory process is based upon a multidisciplinary review of the evidence submitted by drug developers and is heavily reliant on phase III randomized clinical trials. Statistical tests of inference, to which so much attention is paid during regulatory review, can indicate whether observed therapeutic or adverse effects seen in licensing studies are attributable to chance alone. However, these tests do not indicate whether the sum of observed positive effects outweighs a countervailing sum of harms (assuming the harms have been identified). So how do regulators then weigh all of the evidence of benefit and risk to determine a product's overall value? Despite decades of pharmaceutical regulation, there is no generally accepted, systematic method for conducting benefit–risk assessment (see Box 2).

In principle, statistical confidence in estimates of a drug's risks and benefits should also be part of a transparent benefit–risk calculation. The relative uncertainty associated with these estimates should be part of the calculation, as should the willingness of patients or clinicians to assume the risk of harm for potential therapeutic benefit. For instance, when regulators decided to add strong warnings about suicidal ideation in children and adolescents to the prescribing information of selective serotonin reuptake inhibitors (EMEA, 2005, FDA, 2007), some clinicians began to ask whether a potential loss in benefit would result from decreased drug use among populations for whom benefit was still believed to outweigh risk (Valuck et al., 2007). Perhaps the most depressed paediatric patients derive more benefit than harm from these drugs? It is unclear whether or to what extent regulators estimated the forgone benefit as a result of their 'risk management' efforts. It is not clear how regulators weighed various

BOX A2.2 BENEFIT–RISK ASSESSMENT

Definition of benefit–risk assessment

Per the EMEA Working Group on Benefit–risk Assessment, this is a regulatory process of evaluating the balance of 'observed benefits and harms, as well as the uncertainties and risks' associated with a particular product. The EMEA adds that 'There are no standard quantitative methods to be recommended for evaluating the balance of benefits and risks. Generally, the evaluation of the balance relies on balancing as objectively as possible benefits and harms, each consisting of several different events of different importance and estimated with variable precision. The estimation of the balance is often not precise and large approximations are commonly used.'

Definition of risk

'Risk' in the regulatory context describes an effect that is harmful to the patient's or public's health and which can relate to the safety, efficacy or quality of a product. Risks are frequently thought of as product related adverse events, which can be serious (e.g. causing hospitalization) or unexpected (not previously observed). Benefit consists of all the disease preventive, mitigating or therapeutic effects.

Current methods of benefit–risk assessment

The EMEA and FDA currently evaluate the benefit–risk balance through a multi-disciplinary scientific review process for assessing evidence of drug safety and efficacy, as well as other sources of safety and efficacy evidence that stem from manufacturing, non-clinical (i.e. animal) and pharmacokinetic data. From these evaluations, regulators then decide whether to authorize an investigational product for commercial use. No guidance or directive currently exists on how regulators might integrate a product's benefits versus risk for decision-making purposes.

Benefit–risk assessment versus cost-benefit analysis and cost effectiveness analysis

Cost–benefit analysis and cost–utility analysis are two forms of health technology evaluation used by health economists to value a technology, using monetized outcomes and utility as measures. Regulatory health agencies are charged with

---

BOX A2.2 (Continued)

interpreting the evidence of a product's effects (health risks and health benefits) to decide whether to permit product commercialization. The methods of evaluation used in health economics and other decision sciences offer a structured means to evaluate a trade off that a decision maker faces. Yet, in contrast to economic evaluations, regulatory evaluations are restricted to scientific data that are not monetized and which do not consider non-scientific issues such as resource utilization, which are common to economic evaluations. Despite the inherent differences between the goals and current methods used in health economic evaluation versus regulatory review, both involve making and optimizing a trade off. Thus, the models and tools used in economics and other decision sciences could be helpful in making these regulatory decisions more systematic, structured and transparent.

---

perspectives on the value of these drugs (i.e. the clinician's, parents' or children's perspective). A role for basing such decisions in part upon formal evaluation of patient or physician preferences for the benefit–risk trade-off could be explored, for instance, by surveying identified subpopulations to see which are most willing to accept potential risks for potential benefit.

These regulatory scenarios would appear to provide an ideal opportunity for using some of the traditional tools and methods of health economic evaluation such as mathematical modelling and utility measurement (see Box 2). These approaches offer a systematic way of informing decision-makers about the value of a technology. They also permit exploration of a product's value from various perspectives. Yet, in general, regulators are charged with considering only health outcomes and not costs or resource utilization. They must consider benefit–risk in the terms of clinical endpoints and do not attempt to monetize health states such as adverse events. To this extent, new methods or variations on existing methods of health economic evaluation would be needed if health economists are to help inform decision-makers in medical product regulation. This was the rationale behind the OHE meeting.

Given the limitations to the current method of assessing drug benefit–risk, the EMEA's CHMP set up a working group in May 2006. The working group described the feasibility of four different approaches for regulatory assessments (EMEA, 2007a). None of these was explicitly an economic approach; the October 2007 OHE workshop was organized to discuss these approaches as well as what an economic perspective might add. The OHE workshop participants debated whether an economic perspective could help to improve the current regulatory paradigm. For example, can tools commonly used by health economists and other decision science disciplines improve the transparency of the benefit–risk assessment process by explicitly linking how evidence of risk and benefit was weighted in the final assessment and regulatory decision? Whereas the current approach is often accused of applying inconsistent standards for regulatory approval, might new methods bring about greater consistency when defining benefit and risk across a range of products? If a rare adverse event (e.g. severe rhabdomyolysis for a new cholesterol lowering drug) was reported in a clinical trial for two persons out of 1000 taking an unapproved drug but for none among the 1000 on placebo, how would the risk of that event be weighted in the ensuing regulatory decision? How does uncertainty around this risk differ from uncertainty around risks observed for previously approved products of the same indication? How much uncertainty in the estimate of risk versus benefit can stop a product from licensure? What are the important factors in that benefit–risk decision and how are the attributable effects of each factor weighted? Lastly, to what degree does regulator acceptance of a given degree of risk for a given degree of benefit reflect what patients (or consumers in general) are willing to accept? Health economic and decision analytic approaches can address many of these regulatory concerns regarding benefit–risk trade-offs.

Dr Eric Abadie, Chair of the CHMP, set the stage for the discussion and debate of these issues with his opening presentation. He remarked on the CHMP's efforts to improve benefit–risk assessment methodology:

> Today the benefit–risk balance of new chemical entities is based on evaluation of extensive evidence, based on clinical efficacy and safety, but also, at the end of the day, on subjective judgment. This subjective judgment could in fact more or less preclude some transparency and some consistency. That is why we decided to undertake this work – in order to be more transparent and more consistent.

A2.4 OVERVIEW OF NEW APPROACHES TO BENEFIT–RISK ASSESSMENT

Four approaches to aid regulatory benefit–risk assessment were discussed at the October 2007 OHE meeting.

Health outcomes modelling with QALYs

Modelling with quality-adjusted life years (QALYs; see Box 3) involves the construction of a disease-state model that links various health states associated with the disease under consideration (e.g. metastatic cancer, remission, death) as well as the various treatment-related adverse effects. Life expectancy adjusted for health-related quality of life (i.e. QALYs) is used to integrate all outcomes into a single metric. By virtue of constructing

BOX A2.3 HEALTH OUTCOMES MODELLING USING QUALITY-ADJUSTED LIFE-YEARS

The models used in health outcomes research often use the unitary metric of the quality-adjusted life-year (QALY) to compare non-monetary outcomes across different types of interventions. The QALY represents an adjustment to length of life for the quality of life experienced. This measure can be easily adapted to benefit risk assessment by separating the outcomes into expected health improvements with positive QALYs (benefits) and adverse health impacts with negative QALYs (risks) to yield an incremental net health benefit comparing two interventions. – L. Garrison.

Incremental net health benefit (INHB) of new Drug 2 versus conventional Drug 1 can be expressed as:

$$INHB = (E2 - E1) - (R2 - R1)$$

where effectiveness (E) is measured in QALYs and risk (R) can also be measured in QALYs.

Strengths

- Can compare benefit versus risk quantitatively in terms of aggregated QALYs for a population, thereby assigning a weight to each outcome using utility.

- Explicitly considers uncertainty and heterogeneity of preferences across individuals.

- Considers the costs and benefits of gathering additional information (that is, the value of information) where regulatory decisions are delayed or post-licensing studies are mandated.

- Provides a model structure with quantitative parameters that an advisory committee could explore in its deliberations using sensitivity analyses.

Current limitations

- Utility does not usually explicitly capture patient risk aversion.

- QALYs less well understood as a decision-making 'yardstick' by regulators, physicians and patients.

the model, the links among the different health states, the treatment effects considered relevant to benefit–risk, the link between surrogate and clinical outcomes, and the probabilities for developing various outcomes are all defined explicitly. Garrison and colleagues have argued for constructing these models at a population level, considering multiple subgroups and potential losses in health net-benefit due to delays in reaching a decision (Garrison *et al.*, 2007) Such modelling can also inform decision makers about the value of collecting additional information to reduce uncertainty in the risk-benefit decision, by identifying which effects most influence the overall estimate (Briggs 2006). Health outcomes modelling can be seen as an extension or broadening of the incremental net benefit approach, discussed next, to include population-level impacts, such as the health benefits forgone in delaying an approval decision.

Incremental net benefit

The incremental net benefit approach (see Box 4) aims to quantify the difference in net benefit for an intervention relative to a comparator. Data sources and model construction must be justified, just as with health outcomes modelling with QALYs. Incremental differences in outcomes can be quantified in terms of QALYs or in terms of clinical events (Lynd, 2004, 2007a, b) Computer simulations of outcomes can be used to calculate probabilities of an intervention exceeding a specified threshold of incremental benefit. (Lynd, 2004) This can be informative when the threshold is linked to acceptability of benefit–risk, as it can then quantify the probability of positive or negative benefit–risk decisions. Stratum-specific estimates for health outcomes can also be incorporated in the analysis to provide subpopulation level estimates of net benefit.

Stated preference

The stated preference approach (see Box 5) aims to address the potential discrepancy between regulators and patients or clinicians in what is considered to be an acceptable benefit–risk trade-off. Since the public entrusts a regulatory authority to make benefit–risk decisions on its behalf, the regulatory authority is assumed to act in a manner that is consistent with what its constituents seek. However, some would argue that regulatory agencies may be more conservative in their licensing decisions than their constituents might like given the negative attention drawn to regulators by 'incorrect' decisions. This is most evident when patient advocacy groups lobby regulators to reinstate a product (e.g. alosetron, natalizumab). The stated preference approach surveys subjects in order to elicit – hypothetically – the maximum acceptable risk and minimum acceptable benefit of a product. This approach can be particularly useful to evaluate how risk acceptance changes as a function of the severity of harm, or as a function of therapeutic effect size or baseline patient covariates such as age (Johnson & Hauber, 2007).

BOX A2.4 INCREMENTAL NET BENEFIT (INB) FOR QUANTITATIVE BENEFIT–RISK ASSESSMENT

Is this a tool that can help us evaluate whether the benefits outweigh the risks from a regulatory perspective or a clinical perspective? I think one of the key issues is it does make the data explicit and it does make the preference weights explicit and if at any point anybody disagrees with any of the data that one uses in one of these analyses you can change the analysis, you can incorporate different data and see if that changes the outcomes and it does make it explicit. – L. Lynd.

$$INB = (E_A - E_S) - (H_A - H_S)$$

where E = effectiveness, H = harm, A = alternative product, S = standard/comparator.

$$\text{Expected INB} = \sum \text{expected treatment benefit} - \sum \text{expected treatment harm}$$

Strengths

- Utilizes all available epidemiological evidence.

- Can incorporate multiple outcomes that might affect decision.

- Can perform sensitivity analyses on effect of uncertainty in model inputs, including risk and benefit.

- Can incorporate alternative patient-preference weights, including conventional health-state utility weights and generalized preference weights.

- Can produce stratified estimates of benefit–risk (see figure below).

BOX A2.4   (Continued)

Current limitations

• Results are model-derived, and therefore subject to assumptions and to model validity.

• Net benefit may not be easily translatable to end-users (clinicians, patients).

• Weights for outcomes subject to method of ascertainment.

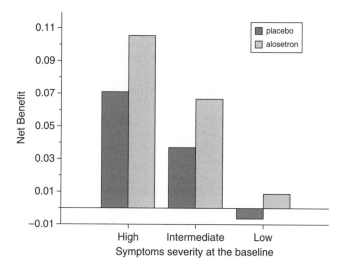

Incremental net benefit of alosetron for irritable bowel syndrome, stratified by baseline disease severity. Treatment benefit is positively associated with baseline severity. Thus INB can also guide regulatory decisions at a subpopulation level of benefit–risk where subpopulation specific determinants of heterogeneity are known.

MCDA

Multi-criteria decision analysis (see Box 6), a tool from the decision sciences, aims to define more consistently and transparently the criteria for technology evaluation (Phillips and Costa, 2007). It provides a systematic group process for identifying attributes of product risk and benefit that are deemed relevant for making a

BOX A2.5 STATED-PREFERENCE METHODS FOR BENEFIT–RISK ASSESSMENT

Quantifying patients' benefit–risk threshold

- Preferences among alternatives depend on the relative importance of attributes.

- Hypothetical alternatives consist of combinations of attributes.

- Subjects state preferences in series of choices involving hypothetical alternatives.

- Pattern of choices identifies willingness to accept trade-offs.

- Statistical model identifies implicit preference weights.

Strengths

- Satisfies the regulatory need to understand patient preferences before the health outcomes of a product are accurately identified.

- Does not require data on observed outcomes. Preferences, not clinical evidence, are assessed.

- Realistic incorporation of non-linear preferences:

  ▶ A given change in benefit is valued differently depending on where it occurs on the severity scale.

  ▶ Conventional health utility is assumed to be a linear function.

  ▶ Risk aversion requires non-linear preferences.

- Provides estimates of maximum acceptable risk, minimum acceptable benefit, maximum acceptable number needed to treat, minimum acceptable number needed to harm, net benefit, net safety margin.

BOX A2.5 (Continued)
Current limitations

- Hypothetical bias: patients may choose differently among real treatment alternatives.

- Measurement error: data quality may be poor if trade off tasks are too difficult.

- Innumeracy: people have a poor understanding of small probabilities.

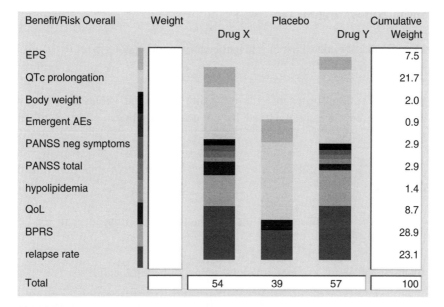

Benefit/Risk Overall	Weight	Drug X	Placebo	Drug Y	Cumulative Weight
EPS					7.5
QTc prolongation					21.7
Body weight					2.0
Emergent AEs					0.9
PANSS neg symptoms					2.9
PANSS total					2.9
hypolipidemia					1.4
QoL					8.7
BPRS					28.9
relapse rate					23.1
Total		54	39	57	100

Risk-benefit functions indicate that population preferences (white lines) for benefit–risk trade offs change non-linearly, based on the magnitude and severity of risks and benefits conferred by the product. Preferences elicited from multiple populations or subgroups can be compared to a regulator's valuation of the trade off (blue line), to ascertain when and for whom the two functions might lead to discordant valuations of overall benefit–risk.

---

regulatory decision. The attributes are weighted by the decision-makers to provide a transparent valuation of various outcomes or product features (e.g. adherence). Because the same regulatory-product scenario can be presented to different decision-makers, MCDA has also been proposed as a way to explain why

BOX A2.6 MULTI-CRITERIA DECISION ANALYSIS

This is a simplification of a part of something that the regulators need to do. It does not give you the answer as to what to do but it can clarify thinking to the extent that you will now find it easier as a group of regulators to agree amongst yourselves as to what to do. It is a constructive model, it is helping people to be clear about their preferences and to construct preferences that they feel will be reasonably robust, can be reported in the public, can be made available – L. Phillips.

Steps to conducting MCDA

- Identify and organize a list of relevant benefit and risk criteria for determining the benefit–risk profile.

- Score the options on each criterion, using numerical values between two reference points and either a fixed, but not necessarily linear, scale or a relative preference scale.

- Assign weights to each criterion to reflect their relative importance in the decision.

- Multiply the options score by the weight for each criterion; sum for both benefits and risks.

- Examine the result, compare the total scores of benefits and risks.

- Use sensitivity analyses to explore the effects on the overall results of imprecision and of differences of opinion about the scores and weights.

Strengths

- Can be used across disease states, treatments and populations.

- Incorporates new data from various sources. Able to incorporate uncertainty.

BOX A2.6 (Continued)

- Accommodates multiple risks and benefits and various comparators. Characterizes objective risks (e.g. mortality) as well as subjective benefits (e.g. health-related quality of life).

- Considers preferences of decision-makers (subjective perceptions of weights) by applying protocols.

Current limitations

- Benefit–risk profiles are snapshots in time: new evidence may demand revised assessments.

- Further efforts are required to develop appropriate scales for the different benefit and risk attributes.

- Resource consuming to develop a MCDA model.

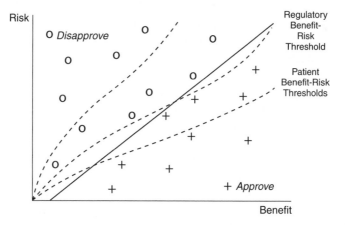

Overall preferences for benefits and risks for a new antipsychotic drug X compared to existing drug Y and placebo. The left column lists criteria: the first four are risks, the next six are benefits. Segments of the stacked bar graphs show the contributions of each criterion to the total weighted scores (bottom row). Weighted preferences are displayed: longer segments for risks signify lower risks; longer segments for benefits signify higher benefits. Judged relative weights of the criteria (right column) indicate the relative importance of the ranges of the criterion scales on which the three options were scored (Walker *et al.* 2006).

different agencies make different decisions, given the same set of data (Walker and Cone, 2004).

Discussion of these four approaches at the October 2007 OHE workshop led to the emergence of three major themes: (1) transparency of benefit–risk assessments; (2) role of preferences in assessments; and (3) the extent of consistency and impact of uncertainty in risk or benefit on decisions.

A2.5   TRANSPARENCY

Both US and European regulatory authorities have indicated that one important way to improve the benefit–risk decision-making process is to increase its transparency (Galson, 2007; EMEA, 2007a).

Dr Abadie provided a working definition of transparency:

> Being transparent means to explain to the outside world how we assess benefit–risk. We regulators have been accused by some stakeholders who disagreed with our past opinions, of being not so transparent. These stakeholders did not understand why we had taken a negative or positive decision.

The proposed methodological approaches address the issue of transparency in benefit–risk assessments from different angles, by explicitly stating: (1) the criteria of risk and benefit that are relevant to the assessment, and (2) how relevant data are weighted in the decision.

With regard to establishing the relevant criteria, it is 'extremely important to describe all potential criteria for benefit or risk that will be used to make a licensing determination' said Dr Abadie. Dr Larry Phillips of the London School of Economics reiterated Dr Abadie's point, 'Whatever you consider to be a risk or a benefit, one must have a fundamental understanding of risk and benefit as they relate to the scenario at hand if you are going to balance benefit against risk.'

Under conventional regulatory decision making, an array of data will be analysed by reviewers to inform the decision. But, as Dr Larry Lynd of the University of British Columbia noted, the conventional approach does not render this very clear to stakeholders. In the case of rofecoxib's removal from the market:

> the conclusions of the expert panel were in fact that the potential risks outweighed the potential benefits but this conclusion was reached relatively subjectively; they did not explicitly quantitatively trade them off simultaneously, but certainly evaluated all the data and made a decision.

Thus, it was not transparent which data were used and how they were used.

Dr Abadie noted that MCDA is an approach under discussion in Europe and that it 'will define the list of benefits and the list of risks, which is one of the objectives that we should have'. Dr Phillips said that 'Multi-criteria decision analysis is a methodology for appraising options on the individual, often conflicting, criteria and combining them into one overall appraisal.' Component criteria are defined through consensus panels of relevant experts.

The incremental net health benefit (INHB) and health outcomes modelling approaches address the transparency of criteria informing the decision. These approaches explicitly quantify the outcomes data that are included in determining benefit and risk estimate for each intervention. That is, the summary estimates of risk and benefit from the model outputs are each composed of various model inputs of probabilities and weights for harms and benefit that should be clearly presented. The MCDA approach uses a consensus of experts to estimate 'preference values' associated with various clinical outcomes. For INHB benefit–risk models, the selection of inputs usually comes from clinical trials, retrospective studies, and patient- or community-reported 'preference' studies, estimating rankings for different health outcomes. It can be debated whether MCDA or INHB modelling is more subjective, as all modelling requires that assumptions be made. 'A virtue of modelling', noted Dr Louis Garrison of the University of Washington, 'is that the reviewers can examine the entire model, so they can see how the surrogate outcomes are linked to the final outcomes estimates of benefits and risks'. Often it is left for the modeller to decide which parameter values to use in the end, yet model inputs should remain transparent, have clinical face validity, and be defensible.

A distinction between the modelling and MCDA approaches can also be seen in how evidence informing the decision is integrated in the final decision. The MCDA approach is driven by expert panel weighting and scoring of the component criteria. In the case of health outcomes modelling, probabilities and weights (e.g. the utility of health states) are obtained from available data or specific studies. Dr Lynd felt that:

> one of the key issues is that modelling does make the data explicit and it does make the preference weights explicit. If at any point anybody disagrees with any of the data that one uses, you can change the analysis: you can incorporate different data and see if that changes the outcome and it does make it explicit.

The criteria for risk and benefit in the stated-preference approach differ from the MCDA or modelling approaches. Criteria are derived from what patients perceive to be clinically relevant. However, the options presented to them in the trade-off scenario are ultimately determined by the assessor. Overall risk and benefit are not evaluated separately and then aggregated, as is done for MCDA and modelling. Rather, they are presented as a composite, a sort of 'holistic approach' in which the overall clinical trade-off is described. An advantage of disaggregating before presenting an intervention's net impact on health outcomes is that, as Dr Garrison said, 'It is important to show the intermediate outcomes before showing the final calculated result because the calculation is complex and may not be very intuitive for people.' On the other hand, Dr Reed Johnson of Research Triangle Institute indicated that the point of eliciting preferences in a 'holistic' manner is to, 'offer people alternatives or scenarios that replicate something that conceivably one could encounter in a real clinical setting and these alternatives consist of attributes or features of particular treatment in this case, and there can be positive and negative consequences of treatment,' which may or may not necessarily be perceived by patients by their individual components but in aggregate.

The proposed methods have advantages over some of the existing approaches used to describe benefit–risk. This is most evident when trying to describe the totality of data or complexity of the clinical scenario. 'The number needed to treat and the number needed to harm – to me as a clinician – is something that I like. I like it because it is easy to calculate, it speaks for itself, and it is increasingly used in the scientific literature,' said Dr Abadie. But, 'one of the shortcomings is that it does not take into account the whole dossier but it is mostly adapted for one clinical trial and essentially for binary endpoints'.

With regard to the stated-preferences approach, Dr Brett Hauber of Research Triangle Institute described maximum acceptable risk and minimum acceptable benefit as 'analogous to the number needed to treat and number needed to harm, except that they are preference-based rather than event-based.' If this is the case, then it raises the issue that stated preference approaches may be similarly challenged in their ability to consider all data that are potentially relevant to the trade-off between benefit and risk. However, the stated preference approach offers the possibility of eliciting preferences that mimic as much as possible real medical decision scenarios, which may not be achieved with methods of assessment that examine the trade-off at the trial-level or endpoint level.

In terms of the transparency of the weighting process, each method presents its own opportunity and challenge. The weakness of the current approach was summarized by Dr Garrison: 'The experts and regulators have subjective and unobservable weights on the pieces of information that they are considering, so their underlying framework is inherently implicit.'

The MCDA approach offers a potential improvement over the current approach in this respect. As Dr Phillips pointed out:

> it incorporates judgements about the impact of data, converting the measured performance of a product, in terms of benefit–risk, into what it is actually valued as. It allows for differential importance of decision criteria, and it is based on a sound theory that only assumes that decision makers wish their decisions to fit together.

However, one potential drawback of MCDA, shared by Dr Abadie and others is that 'the consensus panel assigns weights to each of the criteria that comprise benefit and risk. So, the weight of this tree [of benefit–risk information] is totally subjective.' Yet as Dr Phillips indicated, each method introduces subjectivity into the benefit–risk assessment process, and the advantage of the MCDA approach is that 'it makes the subjective explicit and defendable.' For instance, the modelling approaches and stated preference approach each involve assumptions about what should be included in the model and what should be asked of the patient.

This begs the larger question: if each proposed method introduces its own form of subjectivity, whether it be the inputs chosen for the model or the preference options they chose to elicit, then how do we capture the effect of this subjectivity? Can it be minimized? Dr Phillips stated, 'MCDA or not, regulatory decision makers currently make implicit judgements about which risks and benefits are more important than others'.

Modelling with QALYs uses utility weights derived from approaches such as standard gamble, time trade-off, or visual-analogue scale, which have a number of limitations (McGregor and Caro 2006). As Dr Johnson noted:

> the standard-gamble preference-elicitation format does not reveal anything about risk aversion. Yet risk aversion is a fact of daily life. It is inherent in the way physicians think about prescribing medication and it is inherent in the way patients think about the medication prescribed for them. So it is essential to incorporate that reality in how we evaluate products.

(see Box 5). Dr Garrison agreed that risk aversion is an important consideration but argued that it can be incorporated into the health outcomes modelling approach by requiring a margin of positive expected net benefit or by explicit inclusion in the valuation of health states.

There was concern that the approaches may simply introduce more complexity to the decision making process, and reduce the transparency that each approach seeks to provide. Dr Andrew Briggs of the University of Glasgow, asked that

> we should try not to confuse transparency with complexity. I think you can have a fairly transparent but quite complex model or the other way round ... There are many ways in which we can learn about how better to present our methods and maybe also ask ourselves the difficult question about 'Can we make it simpler without becoming simplistic?

Dr Phillips suggested that simplifying the regulatory benefit–risk decision should not itself be a primary goal. 'Why do we expect decisions about the outcome of that comparably complex process to be so simple that you can reduce it to just a few criteria and numbers to then make a decision? I think the regulators have a complex job and they need models to help them make it simple and transparent; as simple as possible but not too simple.'

A2.6   PREFERENCES

The second major theme of the workshop was that of preferences: Whose preferences matter for benefit–risk assessment? How can we determine whether different perspectives result in different determinations of benefit–risk? In what way are these issues manifested in current and proposed approaches?

Much of this discussion centred on perspective. Dr Phillips asked, 'Whose preferences do we use? Do we use society's, the regulator's or patients' preferences?' The reason for much debate on this topic was captured succinctly by Dr Hauber, who related differences in preferences to differences in regulatory decisions:

> It is possible that regulators' preferences actually reflect societal benefit–risk preferences . . . However, in some cases the general population may be more risk-averse than regulators. In that situation some drugs would be approved that would not be acceptable to the general population . . . Likewise, it is possible that . . . risk tolerance is greater among the general population or among particular stakeholders and there then could be cases where people believe they are being unjustly denied access.

Regulators, as Dr Abadie noted, are grappling with how to better reflect patient preferences. This would entail, 'taking into consideration the presence of alternative therapies and involving industry in the reflection.' This will present a challenge where placebo-controlled trials are conducted since these do not yield direct-comparison data that reflect the actual choices among therapeutic substitutes facing clinicians and patients.

MCDA is one approach for tackling differences in preferences. Dr Phillips stated that, unlike other proposed methods, 'The purpose of MCDA, is not to get the right answer, because when there are multiple criteria there cannot be a right answer. . . It is to provide a structure for thinking, so that a group of people with different perspectives on the issues can use it to construct their preferences.' The MCDA approach can compare and contrast how different perspectives and preferences result in different criteria, weights for those criteria, and resultant scores for benefits and risks. Variation in outcomes is a reflection of differences in perspectives and preferences.

Given the potential for different preferences, how might benefits and risks be valued? According to Dr Phillips:

> We can accommodate the differing perspectives by subjecting them to sensitivity analysis: we can also accommodate uncertainty in that way but if you want to incorporate uncertainty more formally we can also do that replacing some of these value judgments with certainty equivalents in a variety of ways that are all consistent with decision theory.

Briefly, a certainty equivalent is a single-point value judged by a decision maker as equivalent in preference to the future uncertain values that might actually occur.

Dr Garrison noted that we need to account both for differences in both health state preferences and in risk aversion among patients. One point to consider is that bad outcomes may have very low probabilities attached to them. As Dr Garrison emphasized:

> people are generally poor at weighing low probability events, and they are generally poor at predicting ex post utility for a hypothetical state. And their ex ante and their ex post ratings differ. Those of us who advocate these preference-based approaches – either QALYs or risk–risk trade-offs-have some measurement challenges ahead.

For products such as alosetron (for irritable bowel syndrome), which was launched, withdrawn, and relaunched in certain markets, 'we can evaluate the effect of preferences,' Dr Lynd argued. He pointed out that 'Certainly alosetron was withdrawn originally due to the concern over adverse outcomes', and suggested that

> it was likely voluntarily withdrawn based on the risk preferences from more of a societal or regulatory perspective. Then it was reintroduced following the FDA review and a patient lobby where the patients basically said, 'We are willing to accept the risk, we would like to have the drug back, please.' So with the reintroduction, there was a look at alosetron from a different perspective, now more from the perspective of the patients' risk preferences as to how much risk were they willing to accept in order to potentially realize a benefit. Thus, we had somewhat of a measure of patients' revealed risk preferences.

Although explicit regulatory statements declaring risk acceptance levels and the perspective taken are rare, it might seem logical that for severe or life-threatening conditions, or those for which good substitutes are not available, higher rates of risk acceptance may be tolerated for product approval, versus conditions where the opposite circumstances exist.

Through the elicitation of stated-preferences, Dr Lynd felt that one could 'use the same model with different preference weights and see how that changes the result. Wouldn't it be great if we could somehow go back and measure the regulators' risk preference when they were reviewing alosetron?'

In discussing his study examining a hypothetical treatment for Alzheimer's disease, Dr Johnson found that 'Physicians tend to be more risk-tolerant in treating elderly patients. The primary treatment goal for such patients may be to alleviate symptoms. This priority is consistent with assigning a lower relative weight to treatment-related mortality risks for patients with relatively short life expectancy than for younger patients.' This argues the case for exploring the potential for heterogeneity in preferences in different populations and their effect on regulatory determinations.

There are drawbacks to quantitative methods that elicit preferences or utility. As Dr Hauber indicated:

> When we ask people to tell us about their preferences, there is a cognitive burden involved. We have to reconcile the need to provide enough information for subjects to make 'informed' trade-offs with the potential of providing more information than subjects can absorb and use effectively to express their actual preferences. Additionally, most people have difficulty evaluating small probabilities. Whether we are eliciting trade-offs for health-state utilities or for conjoint analysis, there is measurement error which . . . is a direct function of the complexity of the trade-off task. In essence, we want to get as much information as possible from subjects before reaching a point where we generate bad data because researchers have worn people out or made the evaluation task too complex.

Dr Hauber continued: 'The role of preference data will vary depending on the magnitude and character of the societal impact of the decision. Adding to Dr Garrison's comment, quantitative benefit–risk methods offer opportunities to identify those patient groups for whom the net benefit is greatest.' This would help the regulatory process by better defining sub-populations for the product prescribing information, rather than relying on overall population means of benefit and risk. Dr Briggs noted that one could 'make sure that the products get into those patients for whom the benefits are going to be the greatest as opposed to . . . pulling the drug off the market so those who might derive some benefit actually do not have any access to it'.

A2.7   CONSISTENCY AND UNCERTAINTY

Why does consistency matter in regulatory decision making? Dr Abadie noted that inconsistency is symptomatic of subjectivity in decision-making, which led the EMEA's CHMP to form a working group on benefit–risk assessment. Could methods or standards for benefit–risk assessment be applied consistently irrespective of therapeutic class? The CHMP working group's review of EPARs for 33 new chemical entities revealed an inconsistency in how benefit–risk assessment was conducted. The purpose of the alternative approaches now being discussed is to improve consistency. As Dr Johnson indicated:

> making regulatory judgements involving benefit–risk trade-offs more methodical, more consistent, more transparent and more explainable to the public will help manage inevitable post-marketing surprises. When surprises occur, regulators then can say, 'These are the criteria we applied to the available data in making that decision,' instead of saying, 'I wish we hadn't made that decision'.

Consistency is intertwined with transparency and preferences. As Dr Johnson noted, 'The emergence of promising new treatments such as biologics, which also may have potential ill effects, makes difficult decisions unavoidable. Currently, such decisions are made inconsistently across therapeutic areas, regulatory institutions, and clinical settings, so there is a lack of transparency about the relationship between regulatory and therapeutic means and ends.' So, what drives this inconsistency and how can it be mitigated?

A separate question is whether a level of inconsistency in benefit–risk decisions is acceptable to society. For example, it may be acceptable to have a lower risk–benefit threshold for cancer products or treatments for other life-threatening diseases, and higher thresholds for non-life-threatening conditions. Stated preference surveys, value weighting of outcomes in MCDA, and utility-based modelling could permit us to quantify the margin of benefit–risk trade-off acceptable to the public and the clinician community. Where more severely ill patients or those with fewer available remedies derive benefit from treatment, greater risk may be accepted for that benefit, as was the case with alosetron.

Uncertainty, and not only therapeutic-specific idiosyncrasies, may drive the issue of inconsistency in drug evaluation. Different evaluators may have different implicit thresholds at which they approve products. This inconsistency could arise from differences in how each regulator weighs the evidence (e.g. preferences for risk versus benefit), or how comfortable the regulator is with uncertainty surrounding certain outcomes, such as long-term cardiovascular morbidity. This could, in turn, lead to inconsistency in requests for additional phase III or post-marketing trials. There is a need for transparency in how evidence of benefit or risk (or conversely, uncertainty of benefit or risk) is evaluated in order to make the decision process more consistent. Thus, there are issues of consistency of process, by types of products, and across regulators or advisors with different preferences, technical training and experience. While manufacturers and regulators will typically agree upon endpoints and treatment effect sizes needed to establish evidence of therapeutic effect, there is less agreement on how to handle uncertainty in estimates of benefit and risk.

To address this, stated preference approaches allow one to plot maximum acceptable risk and minimum acceptable benefit trade-off curves. One can then analyse the effects of underlying uncertainty if you change the nature of the trade-off, for example, the duration of benefit or the probability of an adverse event. Furthermore, by eliciting the preferences of the patient, the regulator and the clinician, regulatory decision makers can quantify both the magnitude and the uncertainty between these perspectives and how they might affect benefit–risk determinations. It tackles the issue of 'how much are people willing to accept,' a question that is usually fraught with uncertainty. MCDA approaches the issue by allowing different groups to construct their preferences around the clinical decision scenario.

Modelling approaches can address uncertainty by allowing one to explore the effect of consistency through sensitivity analyses of individual estimates (1st-order uncertainty) and of the overall model (2nd-order uncertainty). Dr Lynd provided case studies using alosetron, enoxaparin and rofecoxib as examples. Where this approach is adopted, attention must be paid to the method of utility elicitation, since that can affect the resultant values. Both the stated preference and decision-analytic modelling approaches could address the effects of such uncertainty by incorporating preferences from different perspectives, either directly or through utility estimates derived from different subject groups (physicians, regulators, patients). Additional information on drug risk and benefit can be garnered either through real-world use, or through formal phase III or post-marketing studies. The burden of collecting this information then falls either on society or the manufacturer, which can beget another kind of inconsistency. The health outcomes modelling approach allows one to specify the amount by which variance in risk or benefit estimates must be reduced to ensure that risk does not exceed benefit. Dr Garrison indicated, 'These regulatory decisions are often complicated and include an important question of whether it is the responsibility of the company to fund any of the follow-on studies, or is it society? Suppose a company develops a product that is barely over the risk-benefit bar in part because there is a high variance in the risk estimate. We might argue that they need to fund follow-on studies to reduce that variance.' He noted that value of information analysis, a tool being used increasingly in health economics, could provide a more consistent and transparent approach for determining when additional information should be collected as well as who should pay for it under a consistent regulatory regime.

All agreed that addressing uncertainty in risk-benefit analysis is important but also very challenging given the numerous sources of uncertainty and variability. First, there is the ex ante individual uncertainty of whether or not one will experience a sick health state. Second, if diagnosed with illness, there is often uncertainty associated with the disease progression timing and severity level. Third, if there are treatments available, there is uncertainty associated with the heterogeneity of treatment response. Fourth, there is uncertainty (and heterogeneity) related to individual and societal preferences, both ex ante and ex post in relation to experiencing a health detriment or ill condition.)

A2.8   SUMMARY

Several methods were proposed to improve on current approaches to benefit–risk assessment. As Dr Garrison noted, 'It is probably not reasonable to assume that you would use the same methodology for every product.' Can these methods or combination of methods replace human judgment? Clearly not, as Dr Johnson reiterated that 'Unfortunately, there is no single, quantitative, analytical solution to the benefit–risk trade-off problem. While such methods can help inform and improve the consistency of regulatory decision making, these difficult decisions will always require judgments based on multiple considerations.' We learned from the OHE workshop that the different methods had distinct strengths and weaknesses that lend themselves to being used in a complementary manner, rather than alone or as a substitute for the current process. Regulatory authorities in both Europe and North America, are currently investigating the extent to which these methods can be applied. The May 2008 Annual meeting of the International Society for Pharmacoeconomics and Outcomes Research (ISPOR) in Toronto, Canada devoted several sessions to this very topic. Dr Lynd summarized the vision held by many, 'I think we are going to be working collaboratively to develop a collective group of tools that might be applied in different situations.'

About the authors

James Cross is a PhD candidate in the Pharmaceutical Outcomes Research and Policy Program at the University of Washington (Seattle, USA). His research concerns policy analysis and modelling for regulatory benefit–risk decision-making. He was a fellow at the Georgetown University Center for Drug Development Science and subsequently a project manager at the Food and Drug Administration in Washington DC.

Louis Garrison is Professor of Pharmacy and Associate Director of the Pharmaceutical Outcomes Research and Policy Program at the University of Washington. He currently serves as a director for the International Society for Pharmacoeconomics and Outcomes Research (ISPOR). He was formerly the Vice President and Head of Global Health Economics and Strategic Pricing at Roche Pharmaceuticals.

Office of Health Economics
12 Whitehall London SW1A 2DY
www.ohe.org © Office of Health Economics

Reflection Paper on Benefit–risk Assessment Methods in the Context of the Evaluation of Marketing Authorisation Applications of Medicinal Products for Human Use – Committee for Medicinal Products for Human Use (March 2008)

Discussion of final report by CHMP	22 January 2007
Deadline for comments	13 February 2007
Adoption for release for public consultation	19 February 2007
Deadline for comments	29 MAY 2007
Discussion of revised report by CHMP	February 2008
Adoption by CHMP	19 March 2008

A3.1 REPORT OF THE CHMP WORKING GROUP ON BENEFIT–RISK ASSESSMENT METHODS

Executive summary

The assessment of the benefits and risks in the context of a new drug application is a complex process that requires evaluation of a large amount of data.

Benefit-Risk Appraisal of Medicines   Filip Mussen, Sam Salek, Stuart Walker
© 2009 John Wiley & Sons, Ltd

A CHMP working group was set up to provide recommendations on ways to improve (a) the methodology, and (b) the consistency, transparency, and communication of the benefit–risk assessment by the CHMP.

The group reviewed some well-known methods of benefit–risk assessment, and considered their practical applicability to the CHMP benefit–risk assessment.

Expert judgement is expected to remain the cornerstone of benefit–risk evaluation for the authorization of medicinal products. Quantitative benefit–risk assessment is not expected to replace qualitative evaluation. Nevertheless, several features of the bene-fit–risk analysis methods are of interest, such as:

- The most important benefits and medically serious risks that drive the assessment can be identified more clearly.

- Explicit weights are assigned to individual benefits and risks depending on their importance.

- The strengths of evidence and uncertainty are identified and quantified.

Following this analysis, the working group recommends that the CHMP works in two steps:

1. To revise the current benefit–risk assessment section of the CHMP assessment report templates, incorporating a structured list of benefit and risk criteria and guidance.

    1.1 A proposal for modification is provided (Annex 1). The main features are:

    - To use a structured and mainly qualitative approach.
    - To be explicit about the importance of benefits and risks in the specific therapeutic context.
    - To describe sources of uncertainty and variability and their impact on the benefit–risk assessment.

    1.2 The proposal has been revised based on comments received during the public consultation.

    1.3 The new templates should be pre-tested on a few completed applications for which an assessment is available using the old template. Following this phase, model templates will be produced for testing using a few new applications, at different stages of the procedure.

    Following this phase, the CHMP shall consider the need to seek input of other stakeholders as necessary for further revision.

1.4 Implementation phase: The roll-out of the new templates will be preceded by training of assessors, to be continued on a regular basis, and monitoring.

2. To further research the methodology of benefit risk assessment, involving further experts and assessors.

- To explore further development in methodologies for benefit/risk analysis, including a wide range of quantitative and semiquantitative tools, e.g. by organizing workshops with all stakeholders and specialists of decision-making theory and setting up specific research projects.

- The CHMP should continue to interact with relevant stakeholders on international and European initiatives related to the benefit–risk assessment methods.

A3.2   BACKGROUND AND PROBLEM STATEMENT

The assessment of the benefits and risks in the context of a new drug application is a central element of the scientific evaluation of a marketing authorization application and related variations. The assessment must reach, as objectively as possible, a sufficient level of confidence that a set level of quality, efficacy and safety of the new medicinal product has been demonstrated. This requires evaluation of all relevant data as well as the use of judgement and arguments. Article 26 of Directive 2001/83 as amended states that the marketing authorization shall be refused 'if the benefit–risk balance is not considered to be favourable or if therapeutic efficacy is insufficiently substantiated'. The CHMP is endowed with the task of assessing the benefit–risk balance of new medicinal products. Questions have been raised regarding (a) the optimal methodology to establish the benefit–risk balance of new medicinal products, and (b) the consistency and transparency of the methods used by the CHMP to reach conclusions on benefit–risk.

In 1998, the Council for International Organizations of Medical Sciences (CIOMS) stated that 'it is a frustrating aspect of benefit risk evaluation that there is no defined and tested algorithm or summary metric that combines benefit and risk data and that might permit straightforward quantitative comparisons of different treatment options, which in turn might aid in decision making' (CIOMS, 1998). Of note, none of the main regulatory authorities (EU, United States, Japan) has issued a list of benefit and risk criteria, and detailed CHMP guidance on the principles and methodology for benefit risk assessment is currently lacking. The CHMP assessment report template entails summaries of the main evidence from the different parts of the dossier and sets out the main aspects of the actual benefit–risk assessment. However there is no agreed approach on the methodology to estimate the overall benefit–risk balance or on how to describe the way the evidence is weighed and balanced.

Following the CHMP audit in November 2004 and in relation with OFI No A04010-02 (benefit–risk analysis), the need to improve the methodology for benefit risk analysis has been recognised. The CHMP set up a working group to deal with this matter, aiming to improve the consistency, transparency, and communication of the benefit risk assessment in CHMP assessment reports.

A3.3   EVALUATION OF THE CURRENT SITUATION AND EXAMPLES OF METHODS OF BENEFIT–RISK ASSESSMENT

The working group first reviewed the way CHMP conducts benefit–risk evaluations for the authorization of medicinal products. Real examples of marketing authorization processes and CHMP assessment report templates were examined thoroughly. Indisputably, expert judgement has been the cornerstone of the benefit–risk evaluations for the authorization of medicinal products.

The working group also recognized that a number of quantitative and semiquantitative methods have been proposed to aid the scientific review of drug applications. These methods are designed to weigh all the relevant efficacy and safety data and to incorporate value judgements as objectively and explicitly as possible into a single construct, reflecting the intellectual process of assessing the empirical evidence and uncertainties, accommodating risks and balancing risks and benefits. The working group thus decided to review some well-known methods of benefit–risk assessment described in the literature. The aim of this review was to assess the need for conducting a more comprehensive examination of available methods for benefit–risk assessment, and the need to explore further development in tailored methodologies for benefit–risk analysis.

There is a wide range of quantitative and semiquantitative methods that can be considered for benefit–risk analysis. A non-exhaustive list of examples is referenced at the end of this document. Some of the simpler methods are intended to be used for individual clinical trials, such as for example the number needed to treat/number needed to harm (NNT/NNH) method. More general methods, such as for example the 'Principle of threes' and the TURBO methods have been developed for the reassessment of marketed medicines in case of new safety issues as described in the report of the CIOMS Working Group IV entitled: 'Benefit risk balance for marketed drugs: evaluating safety signals' (CIOMS, 1998). Another method with applications in medicine is multi-criteria decision analysis (MCDA), which is also widely used in business and government decision making. The working group decided to consider this method in more detail (see below). Several methods have also used quality-adjusted life years (QALYs), which is a way of measuring both the quality and the quantity of life lived, as a means of quantifying the benefit of a medical intervention. Finally, besides the few examples mentioned here, there is a large body of research developed by pharmacoepidemiologists or derived from pharmacoeconomics on quantitative and semiquantitative methods developed for benefit–risk assessment. Some of them have been used essentially in the pharmacovigilance field or for purposes of reimbursement. Most of these methods are still in the research domain and their validity and usefulness remain to be tested in various contexts.

The different methods differ in terms of a number of important characteristics in the context of the scientific review of a drug application, such as simplicity of use and the ability to explore different situations and assumptions. Simple methods such as the NNT and NNH as opposed to complex mathematical methods are often preferred by clinicians and reimbursement bodies because they are based on few criteria and are easy to use and to interpret.

More complex methods such as the MCDA, or methods that deal with multiple benefits and risks such as those described by Holden *et al.* (2003), are able to combine judgements and data numerically by assigning weights to the scores given for each of the benefit and risk criteria in a transparent way. Interestingly, MCDA strategies do not simply provide a single score. They provide the degree to which every sub-score and input contributes to that score and can incorporate an element of uncertainty. Many MCDA software tools allow visual and numeric comparison of sub-scores and input contributions for different activities/projects being scored. Similar static and interactive visualizations provide insight into the qualitative nature of the quantitative differences. MCDA strategies are used to inform decision makers of areas worthy of scrutiny and focus and are not intended for a critical use of the score per se. These strategies are also used to gain understanding and articulate the divergence between relevant stake-holders. They can thus lead to a more transparent decision-making process.

Inherently to the practice of epidemiology, many methods can incorporate uncertainties in a formal way. Indeed, the more sophisticated methods incorporate uncertainty about the estimation of certain statistics derived from the data and include the variability derived from the different subjective perceptions between assessors of the importance of different variables and results. For instance, utility functions can be replaced with expected utility functions, which incorporate risk tolerance (Kirkwood, 1997). Alternatively, the inputs can be characterized with confidence intervals or probability distributions and the uncertainties carried through to the method output. The effect is to provide a probability density function for the method score rather than a single value. Decisions can be based on summary metrics computed from this probability density function, for example the probability that the score exceeds a threshold or lies between two thresholds.

One potential issue with MCDA strategies is the lack of a dependence structure among the different variables (which are often treated as statistically independent). For methods that treat all values and weights as independent of each other without an appropriate dependence structure, the results of sensitivity analyses might be of limited value. This issue can partly be addressed by redefining or combining inputs so they are more preferentially independent than when initially created (Keeney, 1992).

A3.4   DISCUSSION

Expert judgement has been the cornerstone of CHMP benefit–risk evaluation for the authorization of medicinal products. Although this is not expected to change in the near future, a number of quantitative and semiquantitative methods designed to weigh all the relevant efficacy and safety data together with value judgements have been proposed. These methods can be useful because:

a) they may stimulate a structured discussion between reviewers on the importance of different data

b) they could highlight divergences between different stakeholders and lead to a more focussed dialogue

c) they could help visualize the strength of assumptions and sensitivity to different weights, highlighting and contrasting the qualitative differences.

General principles of benefit–risk assessment

Under Community law (Regulation 726/2004), in the interest of public health, authorization decisions under the centralized procedure should be taken on the basis of the objective scientific criteria of quality, safety and efficacy of the medicinal product concerned, to the exclusion of economic and other considerations such as 'cost-effectiveness'.

The assessment of the benefit–risk balance should be based on the available tests and trials, which are designed to determine the efficacy and safety of the product under normal conditions of use (Directive 2001/83), and which are generally performed under ideal conditions.

It is important to be explicit about the perspectives of different stakeholders that are taken into account in the assessment of the benefit–risk balance, in particular the perspectives of patients and treating physicians.

Considerations about how the treatment is expected to perform under real conditions of use are relevant in the context of pharmacovigilance activities, for example, to take into account any available information on misuse and abuse of medicinal products which may have an impact on the evaluation of their benefits and risks (Directive 2001/83).

Benefit–risk analysis methods may improve interactions between different assessors and stakeholders

Benefit–risk analysis methods and tools should be regarded as tools to help assessors make benefit–risk decisions. These methods can help to describe and incorporate the uncertainties and variability in perceptions by different assessors and stakeholders. However, these methods should not be used to shift the focus of benefit–risk assessment to overall numerical summaries at the expense of information on the qualitative differences. Each method should be understood as having a margin of error, and users of these methods should have this uncertainty in mind. In the benefit–risk context, excessive reliance on the overall score obtained might amount to making the final decision in one way or another if the score is above or below a predefined threshold. When comparing scores, thresholds can again serve to partition a score difference into ranges with different actions for each range. However, these actions should generally not be decisions on whether to approve a drug or not, but suggestions for the type of assessment activity experts should perform to complete a decision.

The scientific review of a drug application by the CHMP occurs in successive steps as the dossier is updated and issues are resolved during the review. This involves a large number of reviewers and stakeholders. Thus, simplicity of use would be an obvious advantage of any method for benefit–risk analysis. Simple methods do not require time-consuming specification of a complex method structure for every situation, therapeutic area, or even product or indication. However, their simplicity can be a disadvantage in the context of a complex benefit–risk assessment where multiple benefits and risks variables, from binary to continuous, each with different weights and dimensions, need to be incorporated into the method. The danger of methods that are too simple is that of reducing complex issues to over-simplified abstract numerical quantities.

Benefit–risk analysis methods can focus the discussion by highlighting the divergences between assessors and stakeholders concerning choice for weights. The benefit of such analysis methods is that the degree and nature of these divergences can be assessed, even in advance of any compound's review. The same method might be used with the weights (e.g. of different stakeholders) and make both the differences and the consequences of those differences more explicit. If the analyses agree, decision-makers can be more comfortable with a decision. If the analyses disagree, exact sources of the differences in view will be identified, and this will help to focus the discussion on those topics.

Benefit–risk analysis methods can increase the transparency of decisions

An important area for improvement would be to make more explicit the criteria on which a benefit–risk evaluation is being made. Although the systematic use of sophisticated numerical methods may not be necessary, especially when the benefits clearly outweigh the risks (or vice versa), they might be useful in less clear situations. Such methods could allow different assessors and stakeholders to be explicit about the importance given to different data. This could lead to increased transparency and better communication about the benefit–risk assessment process. All these aspects could be reflected into CHMP guidance and templates for the benefit–risk assessment.

The revision of the benefit–risk section of the templates should undergo adequate testing before implementation.

In a first phase of pretesting, different assessors (not involved in the revision phase), should use the revised template for a few completed applications for which an assessment is available using the old template. This should be followed by structured discussion with the assessors, seeking to identify completeness and relevance of the items in proposed in the new template. Other assessors could be called to compare the former templates with the new ones. Depending on the findings of the pretesting phase, it may be necessary to adapt the templates.

Following the pretesting phase, model templates should be produced for testing. The model templates for the benefit–risk section should be tested on a few new applications for the rapporteurs and CHMP assessment reports. Complete assessment reports should still be produced using the current templates. Along with the current templates, the test model templates for the benefit–risk section should be produced simultaneously by both rapporteurs and collected separately. The test model templates should not be circulated to the CHMP or the applicant and should not be considered as part of the assessment report. The collected test model templates should be reviewed at the end of the testing phase by a group of assessors and CHMP members, who should make recommendations for further changes, if necessary. Following the testing phase, the CHMP should consider the appropriateness of any changes to the model templates and, if appropriate, timing for implementation. The CHMP should consider the need to seek input of other stakeholders as necessary for further revision.

The roll-out and implementation of the new templates should be preceded by training of assessors, to be continued on a regular basis, and monitoring.

Benefit–risk analysis methods may be useful beyond initial drug marketing authorization

It is important that the same benefit–risk principles are consistently applied in the pre- and post-authorization phases. Quantitative approaches to benefit–risk might also be useful for the continuous evaluation of products post-approval. The current report is heavily weighted to the initial benefit–risk assessment related to the decision to approve or not approve a new medicine. It is recommended that this work be expanded to include a further examination of the question of how to incorporate post-approval safety/effectiveness data into the risk/benefit analysis (lifetime approach). More generally, benefit–risk assessment is a key component of a number of EMEA activities, and adequate involvement of relevant working parties and committees should be sought (e.g. Pharmaco Vigilance Working Party) as well as sharing of information with other committees (e.g., Committee for Medicinal Products for Veterinary Use, Committee on Herbal Medicinal Products).

Conclusion on benefit–risk analysis methods

Even if no single method is suitable in practice for conducting benefit–risk assessment in the context of the CHMP scientific review of drug applications, there may be a number of theoretical and practical aspects of decision-making theory that can be useful to refine the CHMP assessment, stimulate further work and suggest different approaches. Interest for this field of research should continue and exchange with experts could be sought on a regular basis, in the form of workshops or research projects. Proper validation of any useful methods in the context of CHMP review will be essential. Furthermore, given the knowledge and experience within the EMEA and CHMP, it will be possible to explore further development in tailored methodologies for benefit–risk analysis.

A3.5   RECOMMENDATIONS TO THE CHMP

The recommendation of the working group to the CHMP is to work in two steps:

1. To revise the current benefit–risk assessment section of the CHMP assessment report templates, incorporating a structured list of benefit and risk criteria and guidance (Annex 1).

   1.1 A proposal for modification is provided. The main features are:

   - To use a structured and mainly qualitative approach.
   - To be explicit about the importance of benefits and risks in the specific therapeutic context.
   - To describe sources of uncertainty and variability and their impact on the benefit–risk assessment.

   1.2 The proposal has been revised based on comments received during the public consultation

   1.3 The new templates should be pre-tested on a few completed applications for which an assessment is available using the old template. Following this phase, model templates will be produced for testing using a few new applications, at different stages of the procedure. Following this phase, the CHMP shall consider the need to seek input of other stakeholders as necessary for further revision.

1.4 Implementation phase: The roll-out of the new templates will be preceded by training of assessors, to be continued on a regular basis, and monitoring.

2. To further research the methodology of benefit risk assessment, involving further experts and assessors.

To explore further development in methodologies for benefit–risk analysis, including a wide range of quantitative and semi-quantitative tools, e.g. by organizing workshops with all stakeholders and specialists of decision-making theory and setting up specific research projects.

- The CHMP should continue to interact with relevant stakeholders on international and European initiatives related to the benefit–risk assessment methods

A3.6   ANNEX I

Proposed changes and guidance for the benefit risk assessment section of the CHMP assessment reports

Benefit–risk assessment

The aim of this section is to identify the key observations and the uncertainties that drive the benefit–risk assessment. It is important to avoid unnecessary repetition of technical details already described elsewhere, particularly concerning the methods and the results of the various tests and trials. Here, only the key findings should be briefly identified but no extensive description should be provided.

- First, it is recommended to identify the main evidence and the uncertainties that are considered key for the benefit–risk assessment. In this respect, a list of benefit and risk criteria is provided. The list is extensive, and what needs to be included has to be considered on a case by case basis.

- Second, important benefits, risks are compared to each other in the specific therapeutic context, and a conclusion is made on the benefit–risk balance, explaining as much as possible, principles, relationships between the data and the conclusions, and unsettled issues.

Guidance is provided on how to describe as objectively as possible and how to be explicit about the arguments to support the conclusions. This is done, for example, by describing weights given to the expected benefits and the perception of what are acceptable levels of risk relative to these benefits in the specific context.

Compared to the former template, the main differences are in terms of structure and recommendations to document the subjective judgements explicitly. The aim is to avoid repetition and separate enumeration of quality topics, non-clinical issues, clinical efficacy, and safety results, without clearly stated relationship to the conclusions. Instead, the new structure encourages a description of significant findings and uncertainties in terms of their impact on the assessment of benefits and risks.

Although *the proposed template has been designed with the final CHMP assessment report in mind*, similar templates should be developed for all assessment reports and the section could be updated as the scientific review is conducted.

Introduction

The objective of this introductory section is to briefly summarize the background of the disease and its treatments (e.g. life-threatening versus self-limited disease, availability of treatments) for determining the medical need in terms of benefits and the acceptable risks. This may be complex if the indication includes different situations (multiple indications, populations or dosages) with different benefit–risk categories.

- Briefly state the problem statement (the details should be left to the Introduction section, at the beginning of the CHMP assessment report, see current templates). Ensure that the claimed therapeutic indication is clearly stated. Specify the therapeutic alternatives that are relevant for this benefit–risk assessment, including other treatment modalities, their purpose or intended outcome (a new treatment is evaluated against the background of currently available treatment options and standard of care).

- Discuss in general terms the aims of treatments and attempt to establish bounds of acceptability – namely criteria against which a drug must perform. For instance, define the minimally significant clinical benefits worth detecting. This could be based on therapeutic guidelines.

Demonstrated benefits and uncertainties

The aim of this section is to identify the benefits, and discuss them critically. Only the important results and issues that have an impact on the benefit–risk balance should be described. In addition, unresolved issues or uncertainties should be identified and their impact on the balance assessment should be clearly stated.

There is a primary requirement for convincingly demonstrated efficacy. Benefits are usually described as the positive results for an individual or a population, and the probability of achieving such results.

As a possible guide for this section, consider describing any of the following points. (*This is not a list of mandatory points to be described. The need to discuss or not each point has to be judged on a case by case basis*).

For main trials,

- Describe the main benefits versus comparator, for example, in terms of primary endpoint(s), and main secondary endpoint(s). Discuss and the size of the effect and the statistical evidence (confidence intervals and *p*-values). Consider describing benefits in relevant subgroups (e.g. as defined by age, sex, ethnicity, organ function, disease severity, and genetic polymorphism).

For other benefits, if these are key in the benefit–risk assessment, consider the following

- Describe benefits as observed in non-pivotal trials and extensions.

- Describe other available benefit outcome measures (including patient reported outcomes, patient preference, etc., as relevant).

- Describe the observed patient compliance in clinical trials.

- Describe the potential of the new treatment, based, e.g., on any known benefits for the pharmaceutical class.

Review the results critically. Summarize the most important findings of the scientific assessment of efficacy. The purpose is to describe the strength of evidence and uncertainties. Consider any of the following:

- Discuss the choice of dose, comparator, and endpoints (including surrogates, as appropriate).

- Describe important methodological flaws or deficiencies. Refer to guidelines or scientific literature if useful and describe how deviations from guidelines or scientific advice, if any, have been justified.

- Describe the impact of methodological deficiencies on the estimated benefit, e.g. consider any issues of multiplicity, exploratory techniques, *post hoc* analyses, etc.

- Have measurements and scales been validated? What are the unsettled issues? Is there a need for further studies?

- Describe any negative studies and studies showing no difference.

- Describe the quality of the supportive scientific literature.

- Describe any other issues that may have an impact on the estimated benefits.

- Are the results consistent across different factors, e.g. pivotal trial(s) and supportive studies, all submitted studies and literature, different populations, centres, doses, etc.?

Demonstrated risks and uncertainties

The aim of this section is to give a high level summary of the probability that important negative events will happen. Only those risks that are part of the benefit–risk balance and risks that must be accommodated should be referred to. When considering the importance of different events, it may be useful to refer to the intensity of the adverse event (severity for example), time of the event (onset, duration), and time period over which the probability applies. This should not be a detailed description of the safety profile which is described elsewhere.

In addition, unresolved issues or uncertainties regarding potential risks should be identified.

- Present the most important non-clinical safety findings that have not been adequately addressed by clinical data. If present, refer to key findings for example in terms of toxicity (including repeat-dose toxicity, reproductive/developmental toxicity, nephro-toxicity, hepatotoxicity, genotoxicity, carcinogenicity, etc.), general pharmacology (cardiovascular, including QT interval prolongation; nervous system, etc.), and drug interactions. The relevance of the findings to the use in humans should be discussed.

- With regard to clinical findings, refer to the most important toxicity and other risks that have been described in the clinical safety section of the report, i.e. summarize what were the most important adverse drug reactions (or events). State to what extent these risks are considered to be the major contributors to a risk profile.

- On a case-by-case basis, consider for instance discussing the impact of the following safety aspects:

  – The overall incidence of adverse effects.

  – The most serious/important identified risks.

  – The duration and whether the observed reactions are reversible.

– Possible mechanisms (preclinical data on toxicity and general pharmacology).

– Known and potential interactions.

– Limitations of the data set (e.g. missing data, potential risk factors, subgroups of patients not investigated but potentially susceptible to adverse effects). Discuss the implications of such limitations with respect to predicting the safety of the product.

– The duration of performed/on-going safety studies and evaluate the need of results from long-term studies. Discuss if the safety profile has been quantified and characterized over an appropriate duration of time consistent with the intended use.

– Risk versus standard of care, comparative drugs of the same pharmacological class. Discuss class-effects.

– Discuss the potential of off-label use and risks associated with this use.

• Consider discussing identified and potential pharmacokinetic and pharmacodynamic interactions, potential for overdose, potential for abuse and misuse, potential for transmission of infectious agents, potential for misuse for illegal purposes, potential for off-label use, etc., provided these elements could impact the benefit–risk balance significantly.

The EU-RMP Template may be useful as a basis for the evaluation, i.e. considering the important identified and potential risks and the missing important information. Much of the data needed should be available in quantitative terms as specified in the RMP Template.

Benefit–risk balance

The aim of this section is to compare benefits and risks described above, putting in perspective alternative therapies or interventions (where possible and relevant), and to conclude on whether the benefit–risk balance is positive in the specified target population(s).

The evaluation of the balance should take into account the observed benefits and harms, as well as the uncertainties and risks.

Under Community law (Regulation 726/2004), in the interest of public health, authorization decisions under the centralized procedure should be taken on the basis of the objective scientific criteria of quality, safety and efficacy of the medicinal product concerned, to the exclusion of economic and other considerations such as 'cost-effectiveness'.

The assessment of the benefit–risk balance should be based on the available tests and trials, which are designed to determine the efficacy and safety of the product under normal conditions of use (Directive 2001/83), and which are generally performed under ideal conditions.

It is important to be explicit about the perspectives of different stakeholders that are taken into account in the assessment of the benefit–risk balance, in particular the perspectives of patients and treating physicians.

There are no standard quantitative methods to be recommended for evaluating the balance of benefits and risks. Generally, the evaluation of the balance relies on balancing benefits and harms as objectively as possible, each consisting of several different events of different importance and estimated with variable precision.

The estimation of the balance is often not precise and large approximations are commonly used. This is generally not a problem when the benefits are clearly much larger than the risks (or vice versa). If benefits and risks are expressed in terms of the same event (e.g. deaths) then the balance is also easily quantified. Similarly, the balance compared to other treatments is easily quantified if the different treatments differ only in terms of one type of event (e.g. magnitude of an effect or frequency of an adverse event).

However, when the difference is less clear-cut, and the benefits and risks consist of different types of events, it is important to identify and estimate all contributing factors as precisely as possible, and to describe the importance given to the various factors in as much detail as possible. Also, it is important to assess the impact of any significant approximations on the conclusions.

It is important to consider the different regulatory options for approval (standard marketing authorization, conditional marketing authorization, authorization under exceptional circumstances). If applicable, discuss the eligibility and requirements for these different regulatory options.

Generally, it will be important to describe the following (the level of detail should be assessed on a case by case basis):

- Amount of available evidence to characterize the benefit–risk balance. Availability of comparative data and limitations and potential pitfalls of the comparative analyses.

- Interpret magnitude of key benefits and risks from the perspectives of different stakeholders, in particular the perspectives of patients and treating physicians.

- Discuss the level of risk acceptability that corresponds to the perceived degree of clinical benefit in the specific context.

- State the relevant benefits wherever possible in a way that is comparable to the risks (e.g. potential lives saved as a result of treatment vs. potential lives lost as a result of adverse reactions). In this respect, avoid the use of relative expressions of benefits and risks in isolation. The true medical impact is better expressed using absolute values (together with indication of the precision of the estimates).

- Describe how the benefit–risk balance might vary across different factors, e.g. different patient or disease characteristics. Be wary of uncritical use of overall expression of risk or benefit as these are rarely evenly distributed over a population over time.

- Discuss the sensitivity of the benefit–risk balance assessment to different assumptions. For example, describe the 'worst case scenario' if assumptions are violated.

- The following potential points should be considered, as appropriate. This is not a list of mandatory points to be described. The need to discuss or not each point has to be judged on a case by case basis.

  - When the proposed treatment is less effective as compared to available options, discuss the impact of loss of efficacy.

  - If the balance is assessed to be negative, describe the harm (e.g., in terms of lack of efficacy, toxicity) that the drug might cause if used in the claimed indication (cf. the importance of sensitivity analyses, as described below).

  - Describe how the benefit–risk balance is expected to evolve over time (e.g., when late side effects emerge or long-term efficacy decreases).

  - Describe outstanding issues, submission of additional reports by the company to address those issues, hearings and advisory group recommendations.

  - Make reference to the evaluation of the pharmacovigilance plan and risk mini-mization plan (if any). Describe any communication of particularly significant information to the medical profession, patients or the public that is required. Describe restrictions to product availability or usage.

  - Describe the need for further studies (e.g., the need for studies to improve the benefit–risk balance with further optimization studies, the need for intensive additional follow-up measures or specific obligations, and the need for further development including any paediatric development plans).

  - Describe the involvement of scientific experts, patients, consumers or consumer advocates, and other stakeholders in the benefit–risk assessment.

- Provide a clear conclusion on the benefit risk being positive or not for every claimed indication.

Committee for Medicinal Products For Human Use (CHMP) Reflection Paper on Benefit–Risk Assessment Methods in the Context of the Evaluation of Marketing Authorisation Applications of Medicinal Products for Human Use. Doc. Ref. EMEA/ CHMP/15404/2007

European Medicines Agency
7 Westferry Circus, Canary Wharf, London, E14 4HB, UK
Tel. (44-20) 74 18 84 00 Fax (44-20) 74 18 86 13
E-mail: mail@emea.europa.eu http://www.emea.europa.eu

Commentaries on 'A Quantitative Approach to Benefit–risk Assessment of Medicines' *Pharmacoepidemiology and Drug Safety,* 2007, 16

A4.1 A QUANTITATIVE APPROACH TO BENEFIT–RISK ASSESSMENT OF MEDICINES – PART 1: THE DEVELOPMENT OF A NEW MODEL USING MULTI-CRITERIA DECISION ANALYSIS

Filip Mussen, Sam Salek, Stuart Walker

A4.2 COMMENTS FROM Dr E ABADIE

Directeur de l'Evaluation Thérapeutique et de la Gestion des Procédures d'AMM

1. The importance of rethinking B/R assessment as currently practised

The assessment of benefit–risk (B/R) in the context of a new drug application is a central element of the scientific assessment of a marketing authorization application. It is clear that much has been achieved by better regulation of efficacy and safety issues related to medicines, on both sides of the Atlantic. It has also been said that the benefit/risk balance of a medicine implies a value judgement, which sometimes may be poorly understood from the outside world, essentially the main stakeholders interested by the concept (clinical practitioners and other health professionals, patients and consumers, media). On the other hand the consistency of the assessment of the B/R balance of one particular medicine compared to the others, marketed in the same indication, is paramount. Finally the way the information is communicated has often been criticized. Therefore the rethinking of the B/R assessment balance should be led by three master ideas: transparency, consistency, and communication.

2. Possible advantage of this methodology

Broadly there are two different methods of evaluation of the B/R balance: a qualitative method, and a quantitative one. Some numerical models have been developed. Their aims are to weigh all available efficacy and safety data, and value judgements, as objectively and explicitly as possible. The Multi Criteria Decision Analysis (MCDA) is one of them. Clearly this methodology has some advantages, among them the combination of judgements and data by assigning weight to the scores given for each of the benefit and risk criteria in a transparent manner. It also allows performing a subsequent sensitivity analysis, exploring the dependency of the conclusion on the chosen weights.

3. Difficulties and practical implications

The process of setting up a model is time consuming, requiring building up a complex model for every situation. Moreover there could be significant diver-gences between regulators themselves or between industry and regulators on the choice of weights, although it could be partly solved by sensitivity analysis. Indeed this potential complexity makes the method interesting only for a few cases of assessment of the B/R balance, i.e. those cases that are not easily solved by a pure qualitative value judgement.

4. Personal experience

A CHMP working group has been set up to provide recommendations on ways to improve the methodology and the transparency, consistency and communication of the B/R assessment of new medicines in Europe. The recommendations of this working group have been to use a structured, but mainly qualitative approach. However most of the features of the MCDA models will be integrated into CHMP guidelines and assessment report templates. Furthermore specific training of assessors will have to be performed. The working group also concluded that further research into methodology of B/R assessment was needed, especially through the organization of workshops with specialists of decision theory and regulators from other areas where there may be a greater deal of experience.

A4.3 COMMENTS FROM PROFESSOR GUNNAR ALVAN

Prof. Director General Medical Products Agency Uppsala Sweden

Mussen, Salek and Walker have written two papers on a quantitative approach to benefit–risk assessment of medicines, the first being a method description of one possible strategy to formalize the evaluation of benefit–risk of pharmaceuticals according to an acknowledged multi-criteria decision analysis method (MCDA). The second paper is an extensive case study working through the potential benefits and risks of a new hypothetical and atypical neuroleptic drug.

It is a most pertinent activity for regulatory agencies to make evaluations on the benefit–risk situation for many drugs already on the market. In many cases such evaluations will be open for a very long time period, sometimes up to years and even decades. This work is traditionally done by an *ad hoc* process giving intuitive weights to different facts and then balancing them to reach a conclusion on whether the drug should continue to be used the way it is, whether new complementary information to prescribers and patients has to be given, whether its use shall be restricted or even totally stopped. In the assessment of the causality of adverse effects, successful attempts have been made since long to define when an observed unwanted effect is possibly, probably or with great certainty linked to prior drug usage. The benefit–risk aspects on a global level have not been subject to similar successful and extensive theoretical treatment even if a number of contributions has come during the past decade.

One obvious problem with these evaluations is the lack of natural correspondence between both therapeutic gains and unwanted drug effects. I assume that the usual method to come around this obstacle is to have an iterative discussion where facts and arguments are ground until those in charge of the problem reach a point of view that is commonly accepted. The decisions taken then have to be explained to and maybe even defended against other parties: e.g. colleagues, media, certain interest groups and the public. The understanding of benefit and risk may also be subject to appreciation changing with time as well as located at different times of the life of the patient.

The MCDA has been developed and applied to a great number of fields by its spokesman Prof. Larry Phillips of London School of Economics and he has shared his enthusiasm and knowledge with the authors. The fundamentally evaluative terms embedded in benefit and risk, have to be treated in a justified way in the following analysis. The realm of MCDA provides a way ahead as it allows disassembling a complex problem, measuring to which extent options achieve objectives, weighting these objectives and lastly reassembling the material to integrity. Multiple benefit and risk criteria are taken into account and also the lack of evidence can be handled. Most importantly the method also satisfies the need for making trade-off of benefits against the risks.

The case study shows in detail the work process for a hypothetical drug that is evaluated in relation to placebo and a comparator drug. A wide variety of benefits and risks are brought into the clinical picture and it is all worked through in a confident manner. Among drug advantages are improvement in brief psychiatric rating score, relapse rate and quality of life, a disadvantage is QTc prolongation, which is influenced by increasing dug concentrations secondary to CYP3A4 inhibition.

This exercise is convincingly carried out, but it also shows the laborious character of a full analysis. It is however often experienced that a new method which needs an initial investment in learning and application will pay off subsequently. MCDA offers the advantage of introducing as much objectivity as possible and being able to account for how the value terms are treated. It may be desired to redo the analysis by other workers who may put other weights to the criteria and compare the results with full accountability and transparency. I think the approach is promising enough to justify some full scale application to find out if it adds to practical work in the area.

A4.4   COMMENTS FROM PROFESSOR SIR ALASDAIR BRECKENRIDGE

Chairman MHRA
Risk–benefit analysis.

1. Importance of rethinking risk–benefit analysis assessments as currently practised

The basis of the regulation of medicines and medical devices is the balance of risk and benefit. Although this concept is widely accepted, the attributions of these terms is extremely variable and as the two accompanying papers indicate, the risk benefit balance ascribed by different regulators using the same set of experimental data may vary widely. Thus the aims of the authors to standardize this assessment is to be applauded, although the difficulties of applying the principles in real life situations is not to be underestimated.

2. Possible advantages of the methodology

This is not the first time that such an exercise has been undertaken, as the introduction to the papers indicate. There is thus a clearly perceived wish to standardize this important assessment, but as yet, no uniform agreement how this is best done.

One important application is that such methodology might allow risk-benefit assessments to be performed in a similar way at different times in the life cycle of a drug and also comparing different doses. When a medicine is granted a marketing authorization the evidence of benefit is usually more robust than the evidence of risk which accumulates with increased usage and so the balance may change considerably with time.

An important application of this is to be found in risk management plans which are now an integral part of a regulatory submission. These are living documents, whose content will vary during the life cycle of the medicine. In effect, these plans should summarize what is known of the safety of a medicine, what is not known and what needs to be known and how this might be obtained. As further evidence of safety and efficacy accrue, a risk management plan will alter. It would be of value to investigate the role of the proposed form of analysis in the formulation of risk management plans.

The perception of risk benefit balance may differ between stakeholders. In drugs used to treat schizophrenia, as exemplified in the second paper, the views of the patient, his care and the regulator on this balance may vary considerably. The methodology described could be adapted to accommodate the views of the different parties and emphasize the differences.

At present, one of the less useful parts of a regulatory submission is the Expert Report, whose original aims have largely been substituted by a repetition of industry views of the product and which usually adds little to the quality of the submission. If a standardized assessment of risk and benefit could be substituted for the Expert Report, this might add considerable value to a dossier.

One of the current hot topics in medicines regulation is earlier access to medicines by patients. This has been given various names – conditional licensing, priority approval, accelerated approval – but all signify the earlier regulatory provision of medicines for use than is conventionally practised. The assessment of risk and benefit is a crucial aspect of any such exercise and it would be of value to explore how the methodology described in the papers might lend itself to conditional approval situations.

3. Difficulties and practical implications

The difficulties are both conceptual and practical. Experienced regulators may find a standardised format irksome when they have hitherto relied on less robust and more instinctive ways of making an assessment of risk and benefit.

For such a methodology to work, there would have to be sizeable agreement between industry and regulators on the details of the procedure to be used. Since many submissions are now presented simultaneously to several regulatory authorities, this adds an additional degree of complexity.

None of these problems should prevent further practical exploration and refinement of the methodology described here.

4. Practical experience

I have no personal experience in the use of methodology such as this.

A4.5   COMMENTS FROM PROFFESSOR BRUNO FLAMION, MD, PHD

Faculty of Medicine
Molecular Physiology Research Unit
Laboratory of Physiology and Pharmacology
Brussels, Belgium

These companion papers are a high point in describing the design and potential use of a novel model for the quantitative evaluation of the benefits and risks (B/R) of new medicinal products.

There is little doubt that the current methodology used by regulatory agencies to conclude on the B/R balance of new medicinal products suffers from a lack of consistency and intelligibility. Therefore new methods are needed. Unfortunately, so far there is no validated model for B/R assessment that would suit the needs of all regulatory agencies. Furthermore, one should distinguish between models that would apply to individual clinical trials and more general models.

The paper by Mussen, Salek, and Walker describes an attempt to develop a general B/R assessment model based on the multi-criteria decision analysis (MCDA) theory. This method has been used in other domains and seems appropriate for complex value judgements on benefits versus risks, both of which can consist of multiple items. MCDA operates in several steps, from the identification and weighting of all possible benefits and risks stemming from the clinical trial data (multiple criteria) to their direct comparison in ad hoc scales. The method's rationale and its applicability to the evaluation of medicinal products are well presented by the authors (Part I) and the test application that was performed with a selected expert panel of regulatory authorities and industry representatives (Part II) is very instructive.

I agree with the authors that the MCDA model is relatively easy to understand and use, provided the appropriate software is available and working. Therefore the numerical conclusions that are reached (positive or negative B/R balance) should be easy for everyone to trace back to the original criteria. As a matter of fact, sensitivity analyses based on simulated changes in key criteria are an inherent and valuable part of the model. However, the apparent numerical precision reached at the end of the procedure can be misleading because it may give the impression that the assessment is an objective sum (or subtraction) of numbers whereas in fact the heart of the MCDA model lies in the evaluations of each criterion of the clinical trials (e.g. planned endpoints and unplanned specific risks) on *ad hoc* scales using *ad hoc* weights. These scales and weights have to be agreed upon among the assessor(s). This can be a lengthy process especially if various experts or both regulatory assessors and pharmaceutical sponsors are involved in the assessment. I have participated in one inspiring workshop and in a training session in a small group to learn how to use MCDA for B/R assessment of medicinal products but these efforts were not designed to catch the full complexity of real-life situations. This complexity and thus the true value of MCDA for B/R assessment remain unfathomed.

One paradoxical, and probably weaker, aspect of MCDA-based B/R assessments lies in their true sophistication. On one hand, the model seems to require a complete listing and analysis of all potential benefits and risks, known and suspected, while on the other hand, most regulatory assessors would think that the final B/R ratio is, and should be, driven by a couple of outstanding issues. At the population level, it is extremely difficult to add up, either qualitatively or even quantitatively, a series of minor adverse events or minor benefits occurring in various proportions of the treated population and in various patients, so as to end up with a clear idea of the global B/R balance.

This type of exercise would probably turn out to be artificial. Under such conditions, means should be forsaken and each individual should be evaluated to determine if the treatment is effective. The need for a 'responder' analysis of a given treatment, which is sometimes expressed by regulatory authorities, especially in Europe, points to that direction. It is hard to imagine how the MCDA-based model would help in that case.

An unproved but testable advantage of the MCDA model is its ability to force assessors from divergent fields, e.g. clinical assessors and pharmacovigilance experts, physicians and patients, regulators and pharmaceutical sponsors, to confront their appreciation of key criteria using the same scales. Practical exercises could be run with a simplified version of the MCDA model in these 'discordant' groups to reveal potential gains.

In summary, in my view, it is undisputable that the application of an MCDA-based model to the B/R assessment of new medicinal products would help regulatory bodies display their decision criteria and would thus bring increased transparency to the regulatory decisions. However, until proved wrong, it is possible that an improved structuring of the current, qualitative B/R assessment would reach the same goal with a reduced workload. Efforts should be made in both qualitative and quantitative methods, and the situation should then be reconsidered. Recent discussions between the authors of the current papers and members of the European regulatory authorities have led the CHMP to start to react along these lines. The near future will tell how the imperfect B/R assessment process can be improved.

A4.6   COMMENTS FROM Dr DAVID JEFFERYS

EISAI Europe Ltd

The evaluation of the risk to benefit profile lies at the very centre of the authorization of a new medicine or new medical device and during the subsequent post marketing safety surveillance. The regulatory agencies and their expert advisor committees have to balance the risks and benefits seen in the clinical trial programme and to extrapolate these to wider usage of the product after approval. In the past, expert committees frequently referred to the 'favourable risk benefit profile, or to the benefits outweighing the risks'. On other occasions when a safety issue arose, reference was made to the risks outweighing the benefits. In these instances, many refer to the so called 'risk to benefit ratio'. In reality, it has proven very difficult to balance the full risk picture of a product against its demonstrated and potential benefits. There is certainly no agreed 'ratio'. Indeed, a study of the incidence rates for adverse events or mortality against patient exposure shows wide variation with drugs being either withdrawn or maintained on the market with very different incident rates.

The assessment of benefit is becoming more complex with the development of innovative advanced technologies and with the public and politicians now requiring a detailed explanation to be given setting out the reasons for such decisions. Both the regulators and the health care industries need new models to assess benefit risk. It is against this background that the MCDA approach has to be considered.

The MCDA approach makes possible the integration of different risk propositions and allows for values to be attributed to the different risks and the different benefits. This has a considerable attraction when one looks at the preclinical signals and has to assess these against the relatively small number of patients which can practically be exposed in a clinical trial. The assignment of values allows for the comparison of different parameters which many other models do not.

The ability to undertake sensitivity analyses is particularly valuable. This allows assumptions to be tested and also can reveal bias within a decision. A particular application of this may be in focusing the key question for a hearing or appeal before an advisory committee. This is an issue which the EMEA (European Medicines Evaluation Agency) has been exploring.

The MCDA approach allows cost and economic factors to be added into the assessment. This may be particularly valuable for companies in their critical assessment of key projects. This could be employed most effectively in reaching decisions on licensing or business development opportunities.

A practical concern is the amount of time and resource which may be required to employ the approach for more complex decisions. The decision to approve a new medicine often for multiple indications, involves a wide range of issues. To set up the value system for each of these will probably take a considerable period of time. It is therefore questionable whether this approach can be used routinely by regulators given the large workload faced by most Agencies. There might be similar constraints for companies with large development portfolios. The optimal use of the approach for regulators might be in the determination of whether a product should remain on the market when a new safety signal has emerged. Within industry the approach might be used for difficult and complex projects and could have a valuable role to play in in-licensing decisions.

I participated in the two workshops that were held (in the United States and in Europe) when the model was demonstrated to a mixed group of senior regulators and senior industry personnel. I was also involved in evaluating the model for the European Medicines Agency and more recently within EISAI Pharmaceuticals. My personal view is that the approach is a valuable one which should be more widely used by both regulators and by the pharmaceutical industry. Resource constraints probably mean that this use should be selective and reserved for the more difficult decisions. It is possible that by using the technique even in only a few cases that an organization may find its decision making improved as lessons learned from the approach can be applied to other areas of decision making.

Copyright © 2007 John Wiley & Sons, Ltd.
Pharmacoepidemiology and Drug Safety, 2007 DOI: 10.1002/pds

Forum on Benefit: Risk Decision Analysis – Summary of Discussions and Recommendations – MHRA (September 2008)

FORUM ON BENEFIT–RISK DECISION ANALYSIS

A5.1 SUMMARY OF DISCUSSIONS AND RECOMMENDATIONS

Introduction

The third Forum set up under the Ministerial Industry Strategy Group (MISG) met on 3 September 2008 to examine the tools and techniques currently available to enable the pharmaceutical industry and regulators to undertake formalized assessments of the benefits and risks associated with medicines, their use during the life cycle of the medicine, and what developments were needed to improve on current practice. The Forum also considered how benefit–risk can best be communicated to patients, clinicians and other stakeholders.

Context

There is growing pressure on regulators and the pharmaceutical industry to demonstrate consistency and transparency in the difficult assessments of benefit and risk (harm) that they make. Regulators consider a complex body of evidence, including the

Benefit-Risk Appraisal of Medicines   Filip Mussen, Sam Salek, Stuart Walker
© 2009 John Wiley & Sons, Ltd

epidemiology of the condition, efficacy and safety results of clinical trials, details of manufacturing, pre-clinical studies, as well as effectiveness and safety in real world use including potential long term side effects and patient needs. However, the benefit–risk analysis remains based on expert judgement because there are no agreed methodologies for describing and analysing it. Additionally, what is deemed to be an acceptable balance between benefit and risk associated with a medicine may be different for regulators, physicians and patients when considering different diseases and at different stages of each disease.

The challenges of making appropriate and consistent benefit–risk decisions have been the subject of a number of recent workshops and published papers[1], and some of these were considered in advance by those attending the Forum.

The Forum brought together representatives from a range of organisations with the skills and knowledge to debate the topic, including representatives from the pharmaceutical industry, medicines regulators from the United Kingdom, Europe and the United States, patient group representatives, health economists, statisticians and academia[2]. The specific questions participants were asked to consider were:

- What do regulators and the pharmaceutical industry need to enable them to undertake a benefit–risk assessment, and should both parties be employing the same tools/ techniques?

- To what extent are the currently available tools and techniques mature enough and applicable to meet the need? Are there other tools/techniques that have not been explored?

- Next steps – identify a practical way forward and identify research needs.

- Tools and methodologies for communicating benefit–risk.

A5.2   THE FORUM MEETING

The Forum started with a number of presentations[3] that explained:

- how benefit–risk decisions are currently undertaken by UK and US regulators
- what patients expect to be taken into account in the risk–benefit decision
- various models available to inform benefit–risk decisions
- future research needs.

The remainder of the day comprised a wide ranging discussion of how to respond to the specific questions put to the meeting.

A5.3   HOW BENEFIT–RISK DECISIONS ARE CURRENTLY UNDERTAKEN BY UK/EU AND US REGULATORS

The European Medicines Agency (EMEA) is responsible for coordinating the assessment of most innovative new medicines applying for a licence to market in the EU. Review of those assessments is undertaken by the Committee for Human Medicines (CHMP) on which all Member States are represented. In coming to a judgement about the relative benefit and risk of medicines the CHMP uses a range of methodologies and techniques to assess the information made available to it, but there are currently no methods that can bring together this information in order for a quantitative analysis to be undertaken. In March 2008 the CHMP adopted the report of a working group of the CHMP that set out a number of recommendations to improve the methodology, consistency, transparency and communication of their benefit–risk assessment. In particular, their report aims to increase consistency of approach by those undertaking the review of data through enhancing a template for use by assessors. An associated objective is to make the conclusion on benefit–risk more explicit. In summary, the CHMP's current approach can best be described as predominantly qualitative, where the final decision relies heavily on expert judgement.

The Food and Drug Administration (FDA) in the United States faces similar difficulties in formalizing the assessment of benefit–risk balance. Currently the assessment is a qualitative one, based on data generated from different sources to fulfil different purposes – for example data generated in clinical trials are predominantly intended to demonstrate efficacy whereas post marketing data generation tends to focus on safety issues. The quality of the data varies depending on the source, making it difficult to compare benefits and risks in a quantitative model. Improvements in the evaluation of post-marketing safety data are being discussed. The current focus is on the assessment of benefit–risk throughout the life cycle of the product as this may change, as new uses for the medicine are identified, and it is used in more disparate patient populations. The current FDA approach is similar to that of the EMEA, although they do not have in place a well-developed template such as is used by the CHMP. Work is ongoing to develop a data centre which would aid in analysis of large databases, especially where programming expertise is needed. They are developing a network of epidemiologic data which may be useful in identifying post-marketing safety signals. They are keen to explore the potential use of quantitative benefit–risk models to aid decision makers and to improve communication. The development of suitable models could also in the future facilitate a better characterization of the patient population for whom a medicine will offer the greatest benefit.

In discussing the key issues from these presentations, the Forum agreed that there was pressure on both industry and regulators to be able to demonstrate how benefit–risk decisions were taken. The public, healthcare professionals and public funding bodies all expect to be able to access and to understand how such decisions are taken on their behalf. Greater consistency in approach to benefit–risk analysis is required, and the development of a model or models that generated data in a consistent format and that could be universally applied would be the optimum solution. It will also be important to clearly identify when such models should be used.

A5.4   WHAT PATIENTS EXPECT TO BE TAKEN INTO ACCOUNT IN THE RISK–BENEFIT DECISION

Most patients are unaware of the details of regulation but nevertheless expect their medicines to be safe and to work, and to be provided with information about their medicine to inform their choice. Patients may take a different view from regulators, funders and prescribers of the nature and magnitude of the benefits and risks associated with a medicine, and their views about the acceptability of risk taking may change depending on the disease, its progression and severity. How patients and their views should be reflected in the benefit–risk decision making process is a key question. As patients are increasingly making their own choices (including, for example, by accessing medicines via the Internet), the way the benefits and risks associated with a medicine are explained is becoming more important to assist patients (acting alone or with a healthcare professional) to make informed choices about their treatment.

The Forum acknowledged that although patient involvement in regulatory decision making was growing, it is still often tokenistic and takes little account of the need to present materials in a non-technical way that facilitates their contribution to the debate. The regulator's terminology of "risk" and "benefit" can be unhelpful in making people aware of what they can expect from a medicine. Patient Reported Outcomes (PROs) could become a powerful element of ongoing assessments of benefit and risk if they could properly capture patients' attitudes towards these issues.

A5.5   TECHNIQUES FOR IMPROVING BENEFIT–RISK ASSESSMENT

A number of techniques exist, including those used in other sectors, which may inform an approach to benefit–risk analysis in the medicines field. The benefits and disadvantages of the use of quality adjusted life years (QALY)-based modelling, Incremental Net Health Benefit and Stated Preferences for Risk Benefit were discussed. All these methodologies go beyond purely qualitative descriptions of risks and benefits and can assist in the amalgamation of benefit and risk data to produce a net outcome figure to support decision making. However, in any model that combines benefits and risks to calculate an outcome, it is important to ensure that the methodologies are fully understood by all those involved in making the decision and fully accepted by those affected by the decision. Although such tools offer regulators information, and the opportunity to be more transparent and consistent in decision-making, in the end, the judgement as to whether to issue a licence is still a matter of judgement by the regulator.

Multi-criteria decision analysis was presented as a further methodology that has relevance for benefit–risk decision analysis. The technique provides a way to appraise options on individual, conflicting criteria and combine them into one overall appraisal and has been used for a number of years in other sectors. It provides a structure for thinking so that a group of people with different perspectives on the relative balance of benefits and risks can use it to construct their preferences. In theory, any aspect of the regulatory assessment can be included in the model, not only data on outcomes. Computer software is developed for data analysis which can then be presented in a range of ways to assist experts to take better informed judgements.

The Forum noted the similarities between the various models that were presented, and concluded that it would be preferable to focus on the process required rather than on the models themselves. It was agreed that identifying the key criteria to input to any model to be adopted would be critical to its success. It was also agreed that better ways were needed to assess harms. Once the key criteria have been identified, these would need to be weighted and combined. Any model would also need to reflect patients' and broader society's values and be capable of demonstrating to patients and the public how the model is used to inform decisions. Practical examples of applying models to applications.

Several case studies were presented and discussed. The principles of Bayesian statistics and the pros and cons of available methodologies including Number Needed to Treat, incremental net benefit and QALY were explored. In particular these presentations suggest that there is currently no universal solution to the problem of assessing benefit–risk for a given product, but there are models currently available that warrant further exploration. There is also an issue as to whether decisions taken currently take account of patients' preferences. One of the difficulties is deciding how much weight to put on, for example, rare events that are devastating for the person who experiences it but will not rank highly in a "harm" section in a quantitative benefit–risk evaluation. There is scope for improved data presentation, communication between regulatory bodies and transparency of regulatory decisions, even if, at the end of the process, expert judgement, rather than quantitative methodologies, has to remain the cornerstone of regulatory decision making for the foreseeable future.

The Forum agreed that a more formal process of decision analysis would be of value to regulators, and that the communication to patients about how decisions had been taken was essential if they were to engage in a meaningful debate about treatment options. The challenges of applying models to ongoing post-licensing decision analysis, where small serious risks can have a disproportionate influence were acknowledged.

Quantitative methods may better inform the use of available regulatory tools for safety issues emerging post-licensing.

A5.6   FUTURE DIRECTIONS/RESEARCH NEEDS

CMR International had conducted a survey of companies and regulators to identify research needs for benefit–risk assessment which identified a number of current barriers to developing an accepted framework. In summary, there was concern expressed that formalized frameworks minimized the importance of clinical judgement and decision making and lacked pragmatism, that there was no globally recognized approach to benefit–risk assessment, that there was a lack of experience in using such models and concerns about validation and consistency, that some models tended to be complex, inflexible and added complexity to the decision making process.

CMR International held a workshop in June 2008[4] to consider whether a global framework for assessing benefit–risk was achievable, examining the opportunities and barriers to such an initiative, and defining the essential elements to be taken into account by both companies and regulators in defining the benefit–risk balance through-out the lifecycle of a medicine. In summary, the workshop proposed:

- development of a common lexicon to establish terminology and definitions

- further development of framework comprising safety and efficacy parameters developed by the workshop, involving various stakeholders and using a case study approach

- a pilot project with case studies to test the framework among different stakeholders

- a comparative study of current regulatory review templates to improve the consistency and value of benefit–risk assessment

- consider the value of this initiative for those involved in health technology assessments

- further work on applying a benefit–risk framework to different stages of a product's life cycle and integration into risk management plans and on finding ways effectively to communicate benefit–risk decisions to the public.

The Forum agreed that a way to drive this agenda forward would be to establish a leadership group to bring together those with relevant knowledge and expertise. Such a group might usefully comprise CHMP and FDA representatives with invited expert membership, including health economists and the industry. Because of the acknowl-edged need for transparency in decision making the group should include experts who can advise on communicating benefit–risk decisions. The Forum also recognized that the group would face significant challenges in developing a framework that had credibility and the confidence of both regulators and industry and that also took account of cultural differences. It may not be appropriate to focus on a single model. Although there were existing mechanisms for taking forward joint industry/regulator initiatives, the Forum felt that on balance a newly created specifically focused group may make quicker progress on this issue.

Against the background of the presentations the meeting considered the following specific questions:

What do regulators and the pharmaceutical industry need to enable them to undertake a benefit–risk assessment, and should both parties be employing the same tools/ techniques?

The Forum concluded that there are models currently available that could be tested for performance in a formalised framework for benefit–risk decision analysis, and that the same methodologies should be used by industry and regulators. Agreement on the core sets of values to be used and use of common terminology will be important in ensuring consistency of application. Such methodologies could also underpin health technology assessments in the future, although the assessments should continue to be separately undertaken. The Forum recognised that regulatory decisions are complex and multi-factorial in nature and that the weighting given to benefits, risks and other regulatory considerations will differ from indication to indication and, potentially, from product to product.

To what extent are the currently available tools and techniques mature enough and applicable to meet the need? Are there other tools/techniques that have not been explored?

The Forum concluded that there is currently no one model available to apply in the medicines field, and that a framework for benefit–risk analysis was needed within which different models might be examined. Work in other sectors such as the aircraft industry, sectors dealing with environmental and major chemical hazards could usefully be further explored in establishing suitable models. Engineering consultant companies in particular have devised methods for identifying and analysing complex people-technology interactions and for communicating risk in ways that can be understood. Mathematical models and analyses that include probabilistic approaches to population modelling (e.g. Monte Carlo simulation) are developed and there is some experience both with their use, (e.g. food additives/contaminant experts and food manufacturers) and with explaining these methodologies to non-experts. The Forum also recognized that finding a model that will allow the various data ('real world data' – not just data from clinical trials, and including data on benefit) to be brought together for analysis and interpretation – and ultimately communication – will be challenging. The Forum also noted that an additional resource will shortly be available via the Department of Health's Research Capability Programme, providing access to drug registries linked to full NHS clinical records. The EMEA's initiative to develop a template to improve consistency of approach to decision making is welcome and would be a useful contribution in taking the work forward.

A5.7   NEXT STEPS – IDENTIFY A PRACTICAL WAY FORWARD AND IDENTIFY RESEARCH NEEDS

The Forum concluded that if work to take this initiative forward is to be effective it needs to engage key sectors of the regulatory community (EMEA, FDA) and industry. There was support for an analysis of a number of previous benefit–risk decisions as a means of identifying how an outcome was reached, or to taking an agreed and more structured and consistent approach to the benefit–risk analysis in a number of new products. The EMEA's work on developing a template to improve consistency of approach to decision making would represent a significant contribution. The Forum also supported an incremental approach to the adoption of a formal benefit–risk decision model, to be developed and tested alongside current methods. In the longer term, the need better to quantify benefit and risk will require decisions to be taken on what information will be required at an early stage of the development of a drug, and this in turn will inform the drug development pathway.

A5.8   TOOLS AND METHODOLOGIES FOR COMMUNICATING BENEFIT–RISK

The Forum noted that most patients had little understanding that taking medicines involved an element of risk as well as potential benefit – and that most expected those benefits to be significant. Media stories have contributed to the hype associated with medicines. A better way to explain and quantify benefit and risk must be found. Terms such as 'benefits are marginal' are unhelpful in communicating, and use of improved data displays and mathematical modelling may assist in better quantifying messages to patients. An examination of past failures in communication may demonstrate how we can improve the messages that we use.

A5.9   CONCLUSIONS

In closing the meeting, the chairman concluded that.

• There is an enthusiasm for establishing formal mechanisms for benefit–risk decision analysis to contribute to the decision-making process.

- Development of a common lexicon of terminology is essential.

- A framework for benefit–risk assessment is needed, within which different models can be applied.

- An agreed framework would improve the underlying science of drug development.

- We should learn from models in use in other sectors, and ensure that the patient's view is taken into account.

- Different models will be needed for different situations.

- A group (including crucially the EMEA and FDA) with appropriate expertise and enthusiasm should be established to develop a pilot in benefit–risk decision analysis, drawing on work already underway in the medicines field but also considering the value and relevance of methodologies and tools in use in other sectors.

- The importance of improving transparency of decision making and finding ways better to communicate benefit–risk decisions to patients must not be overlooked.

Notes

1. *OHE briefing – Challenges and Opportunities for Improving Benefit-Risk Assessment of Pharmaceuticals from an Economic Perspective*
   Report of the Workshop organized by the CMR International Institute for regulatory Science: Benefit–Risk Assessment Model for Medicines: Developing a Structured Approach to Decision Making
   Assessing a Structured Quantitative Health Outcomes Approach to Drug Risk–Benefit Analysis (Louis P. Garrison Jr, Adrian Towse and Brian W Bresnahan)
   Current Assessment of Risk-Benefit by regulators: Is it Time to introduce Decision Analyses? (D.A. Hughes, A.M. Bayoumi and M. Pirmohamed)
   Quantitative Decision Analysis: A Work in Progress (R. Temple)
   EMEA Reflection Paper on Benefit-Risk Assessment Methods in the Context of the Evaluation of Marketing Authorisation Applications of Medicinal Products for Human Use
2. A list of participants at the Forum on 3 September 2008 are published alongside this report.
3. Copies of all the presentations made to the Forum are published alongside this report.
4. CMR International report: *Measuring benefit and Balancing Risk: Strategies for the benefit–risk assessment of new medicines in a risk-averse environment*.

References

Adis International (2009) *Drug safety*, http://pt.wkhealth.com/pt/re/drs/home.htm (accessed 4 February 2009).

Alexander, T. (2002). Risks should be balanced with benefits [rapid responses]. *British Medical Journal*, 324, eletters.

Andrews E. and Dombeck M. (2004) The role of scientific evidence of risks and benefits in determining risk management policies for medications. *Pharmacoepidemiology and Drug Safety*, **13**, 599–608.

Anello, C. and O'Neill, R.T. (1996). Does research synthesis have a place in drug regulatory policy? Synopsis of issues: assessment of safety and post-marketing surveillance. *Clinical Research & Regulatory Affairs*, **13**, 13–21.

Arlett, P. (2001) Risk benefit assessment. *Pharmaceutical Physician*, **12**, 12–17.

Asscher, A.W. (1986) Strategy of risk-benefit analysis, in *Iatrogenic Diseases*, 3rd edn (eds P.F. D'Arcy and J.P. Green), Oxford University Press, New York.

Bass, R. (1987) Risk-benefit decisions in product license applications, in *Medicines and Risk/Benefit Decisions* (eds S.R. Walker and A.W. Asscher), MTP Press Limited, Lancaster, pp. 127–34.

Beckmann, J. (1999) Basic aspects of risk-benefit analysis. *Seminars in Thrombosis and Hemostasis*, **25**, 89–95.

Beermann, B. (2002) Communication of the benefit–risk assessment to patients: viewpoint of a health authority [presentation]. Drug Information Association Annual Euromeeting 2002, March 6 2002, Basel, Switzerland. http://www.diahome.org/DIAHome/ (accessed 19 March 2009).

Belsey, J. (2001) Reconciling effectiveness and tolerability in oral triptan therapy: a quantitative approach to decision making in migraine management. *Journal of Clinical Research*, **4**,105–25.

Belton, V. and Stewart, T.J. (2002) *Multiple Criteria Decision Analysis: an Integrated Approach*, Kluwer Academic Publishers, Boston/Dordrecht/London.

Bjornson, D.C. (2004) Interpretation of drug risk and benefit: individual and population perspectives (2004). *Annals of Pharmacotherapy*, **38**, 694–9.

Bjornsson, T.D. (1997) A matrix method for the evaluation of therapeutic agents: a framework based on disease process-oriented mechanisms of drug action and their effectiveness. *Drug Information Journal*, **31**, 105–10.

Boada, J.N., Boada, C., García-Sáiz, M., *et al.* (2008) Net Efficacy adjusted for risk (NEAR): a simple procedure for measuring risk:benefit balance. PloS ONE, **3**, e3580.

Bombardier, C., Laine, L., Reicin, A., *et al* (2000) Comparison of upper gastrointestinal toxicity of rofecoxib and naproxen in patients with rheumatoid arthritis. *New England Journal of Medicine*, **343**, 1520–8.

Bowen, A.J. (1993) Benefit/risk assessment: perspective of a patient advocate. *Drug Information Journal*, **27**, 1031–5.

Briggs, A., Sculpher M. and Claxton, K. (2006) *Decision Modeling for Health Economic Evaluation*. Oxford University Press, New York.

Brimblecombe, R.W. (1987) Risk-benefit decisions in human administration, in *Medicines and Risk/Benefit Decisions* (eds S.R. Walker and A.W. Asscher), MTP Press Limited, Lancaster, pp. 115–22.

Brown, J., Chapman, S. and Lupton, D. (1996) Infinitesimal risk as a public health crisis: news media coverage of a doctor–patient HIV contact tracing investigation. *Social Science & Medicine*, **43**, 1685–95.

Brunet, P. (1999) *Dictionary of the main reference terms: pharmaceutical law in the European Union; medicinal products for human use*, Editions de Santé, Paris.

Burley, D.M. (1988) The rise and fall of thalidomide. *Pharmaceutical Medicine*, **3**, 231–7.

Caldwell, D.M., Ades, A.E. and Higgins, J.P.T. (2005) Simultaneous comparison of multiple treatments: combining direct and indirect evidence. *British Medical Journal*, **331**, 897–900.

Califf, R.M. (2004) Benefit the patient, manage the risk: a system goal. *Pharmacoepidemiology and Drug Safety*, **13**, 269–76.

Califf RM, for the CERTs Benefit Assessment Workshop Participants (2007) Benefit assessment of therapeutic products: the Centers for Education and Research on Therapeutics. *Pharmacoepidemiology and Drug Safety*, **16**, 5–16.

Cheung, B.M.Y. and Kumana, C.R. (2001) Should decisions on treatment be based on absolute benefit rather than absolute risk? *New Zealand Medical Journal*, **114**, 214–15.

Chuang-Stein, C. (1994) A new proposal for benefit-less-risk analysis in clinical trials. *Controlled Clinical Trials*, **15**, 30–43.

Chuang-Stein, C. (1999) The role and analysis of benefit and risk in the development of new drugs, in *The Benefit/Risk Ratio: a Handbook for the Rational use of Potentially Hazardous Drugs* (eds H.C. Korting and M. Schäfer-Korting M), CRC Press, Boca Raton FL, pp. 1–10.

Chuang-Stein, C., Entsuah, R. and Pritchett, Y. (2008) Measures for conducting comparative benefit:risk assessment. *Drug Information Journal*, **42**, 223–33.

CIOMS Working Group III (1995) *Guidelines for Preparing Core Clinical Safety Information on Drugs*. CIOMS, Geneva.

CIOMS Working Group IV (1998) *Benefit–risk Balance for Marketed Drugs: Evaluating Safety Signals*. CIOMS, Geneva.

Clemen, R.T. (1996) *Making Hard Decisions: an Introduction to Decision Analysis*, 2nd edn, Duxbury Press, Pacific Grove.

Cocchetto, D.M. and Nardi, R.V. (1986) Benefit–risk assessment of investigational drugs: current methodology, limitations, and alternative approaches. *Pharmacotherapy*, **6**, 286–303.

Cohen, J.T. and Neumann, P.J. (2007) What's more dangerous, your aspirin or your car? Thinking rationally about drug risks (and benefits). *Health Affairs*, **26**, 636–46.

Committee for Medicinal Products (1997a) Note for guidance on medicinal products in the treatment of Alzheimer's disease, European Medicines Evaluation Agency, London. http://www.emea.europa.eu (accessed 7 April 2009).

Committee for Medicinal Products (1997b) Note for guidance on the investigation of drug interactions, European Medicines Evaluation Agency, London. Available from http://www.emea.europa.eu (accessed 7 April 2009).

Committee for Medicinal Products (1998) Points to consider on clinical investigation of medicinal products used in the treatment of osteoarthritis, European Medicines Evaluation Agency, London. http://www.emea.europa.eu (accessed 7 April 2009).

Committee for Medicinal Products (1999) Note for guidance on clinical investigation of medicinal products in the treatment of cardiac failure, European Medicines Evaluation Agency, London. http://www.emea.europa.eu (accessed 7 April 2009).

Committee for Medicinal Products (2003a) Note for guidance on evaluation of anticancer medicinal products in man, European Medicines Evaluation Agency, London. http://www.emea.europa.eu (accessed 7 April 2009).

Committee for Medicinal Products (2003b) Points to consider on clinical investigation of medicinal products other than NSAIDs for treatment of rheumatoid arthritis, European Medicines Evaluation Agency, London. http://www.emea.europa.eu (accessed 7 April 2009).

Committee for Medicinal Products (2003c) Note for guidance on clinical investigation of medicinal products in the treatment of lipid disorders. European Medicines Evaluation Agency, London. http://www.emea.europa.eu (accessed 7 April 2009).

Committee for Human Medicinal Products (2004) Reflection paper on the regulatory guidance for the use of health-related quality of life (HRQL) measures in the evaluation of medicinal products. European Medicines Agency, London. http://www.emea.europa.eu (accessed 7 April 2009).

Committee for Human Medicinal Products (2008) European Public Assessment Report for Avandia, European Medicines Evaluation Agency, London. http://www.emea.europa.eu (accessed 7 April 2009).

Conaway, M.R. and Petroni, G.R. (1996) Designs for phase II trials allowing for a trade-off between response and toxicity. *Biometrics*, **52**,1375–86.

Costantino, J.P. (2001) Benefit/risk assessment of SERM therapy: clinical trial versus clinical practice settings. *Annals of the New York Academy of Sciences*, **949**, 280–5.

Council for International Organizations of Medical Sciences IV Working Group (1998) *Benefit–Risk Balance for Marketed Drugs: Evaluating Safety Signals*. World Health Organization, Geneva.

Council of the European Union (2003) Amended proposal for a Directive of the European Parliament and of the Council amending Directive 2001/83/EC on the Community code relating to medicinal products for human use. DG C I; 2003 June 12. File no. 10450/03.

Cromie, B.W. (1987) Risk-benefit decisions in product license applications, in *Medicines and Risk/Benefit Decisions* (eds S.R. Walker and A.W. Asscher), MTP Press Limited, Lancaster, pp. 135–6.

CropLife International (1997) Some aspects of benefit: risk evaluations in the registration of pesticides, 1 May 1997. Available from http://www.croplife.org (accessed 19 March 2009).

Cuervo, L.G. and Clarke, M. (2003) Balancing benefits and harms in health care: we need to get better evidence about harms. *British Medical Journal*, **327**, 65–6.

Danjoh, K. (1999) Thinking globally: product development, registration, and marketing in the new millennium. *Drug Information Journal*, **33**, 327–32.

Dawes, R., Faust, D. and Meehl, P.E. (1989) Clinical versus actuarial judgement. *Science*, **243**, 1668–74.

Department of Transport, Local Government and the Regions (2000) Multi Criteria Analysis: a Manual. Office of the Deputy Prime Minister. Available from http://www.communities. gov.uk/publications/corporate/multicriteriaanalysismanual (accessed 19 March 2009).

Detsky, A.S., Naglie, G., Krahn, M.D., *et al.* (1997) Primer on medical decision analysis: part 1 – getting started. *Medical Decision Making*, **17**, 123–5.

Dickinson, D. and Raynor, T.D.K. (2003) Ask the patients – they may want to know more than you think. *British Medical Journal*, **327**, 861.

Djulbegovic, B., Hozo, I., Fields, K.K. and Sullivan, D. (1998) High-dose chemotherapy in the adjuvant treatment of breast cancer: benefit/risk analysis. *Cancer Control*, **5**, 394–405.

Dowie, J. (1996a) 'Evidence-based', 'cost-effective' and 'preference-driven' medicine: decision analysis based medical decision making is the pre-requisite. *Journal of Health Services Research and Policy*, **1**, 104–13.

Dowie, J. (1996b) The research – practice gap and the role of decision analysis in closing it. *Health Care Analysis*, **4**, 5–18.

Dujovne, C.A. (2002) Side effects of statins: hepatitis versus 'transaminitis' – myositis versus 'CPKitis. *American Journal of Cardiology*, **89**, 1411–13.

Edwards A, Elwyn G, Mulley A (2002). Explaining risks: turning numerical data into meaningful pictures. *British Medical Journal*; **324**:827–830

Edwards, R. and Hugman, B. (1997) The challenge of effectively communicating risk-benefit information. *Drug Safety*, **17**, 216–27.

Edwards, R., Wiholm, B.-E. and Martinez, C. (1996) Concepts in risk–benefit assessment. A simple merit analysis of a medicine? *Drug Safety*, **15**, 1–7.

Electronic Medicines Compendium (2004) [Database on the Internet]. Datapharm Communications Ltd. http://emc.medicines.org.uk (accessed 20 March 2009).

Elwyn, G., Edwards, A. and Britten, N. (2003) 'Doing prescribing': how doctors can be more effective. *British Medical Journal*, **327**, 864–7.

Eriksen, S. and Keller, L.R. (1993) A multiattribute-utility-function approach to weighing the risks and benefits of pharmaceutical agents. *Medical Decision Making*, **13**, 118–25.

Ernst, E. and Resch, K.L (1996) Risk–benefit ratio or risk–benefit nonsense? *Journal of Clinical Epidemiology*, **49**, 1203–4.

European Commission (1999) A guideline on summary of product characteristics (final, revision 0). Enterprise Directorate General, Unit F2; December 1999. http://ec.europa.eu/ enterprise/ (accessed 6 April 2009).

European Commission (2004) Commission proposes regulation aimed at promoting medicines for children [press release]. Enterprise Directorate General, Unit F2; 2004. http:// ec.europa.eu/enterprise/ (accessed 6 April 2009).

European Council Regulation (EEC) No 2309/93. Community procedures for the authorisation and supervision of medicinal products for human and veterinary use and establishing a European gency for the Evaluation of Medicinal Products, 22 July 1993.

European Council Regulation (EC) No 726/2004. *Community procedures for the authorisation and supervision of medicinal products for human and veterinary use and establishing a European Medicines Agency*, 31 March 2004.

European Medicines Agency (2004) Guidance document; (co-)rapporteur day 70 critical assessment report. Revision 1. The European Medicines Agency; 2004 September. http:// www.emea.europa.eu (accessed 6 April 2009).

European Medicines Agency (2007a) *European Medicines Agency finalises review of antidepressants in children and adolescents.* EMEA/CHMP/128918/2005corr. 25 April 2005, London UK.

European Medicines Agency (2007b) *Report of the CHMP Working Group on Benefit–risk Assessment Models and Methods.* EMEA/CHMP/15404/2007. 19 January 2007, London UK.

European Medicines Agency. *EPARs for authorised medicinal products for human use.* London. http://www.emea.europa.eu/htms/human/epar/eparintro.htm (accessed March 22, 2009).

European Parliament and Council of the European Union. Parliament Directive No. 2001/83/EC. *The Community code relating to medicinal products for human use.* 6 November 2001.

Evans, S. (2008) Special section: benefit:risk evaluation in clinical trials. *Drug Information Journal*, **42**, 221.

FDA (1998) US Food and Drug Administration. *Guidance for Industry: Providing clinical evidence of effectiveness*, May 1998, Rockville, MD. www.fda.gov/CDER/GUIDANCE/1397fnl.pdf (accessed 22 March 2009).

FDA (2007) *FDA proposes new warnings about suicidal thinking, behavior in young adults who take antidepressant medications.* May 2007 Rockville, MD. http://www.fda.gov/bbs/topics/NEWS/2007/NEW01624.html (accessed March 23 2009).

Federal Food, Drug and Cosmetic Act (1997) Chapter 5, subchapter A drugs and devices, section 505.355, paragraph d (amended by the 1997 FDA Modernization Act). http://www.fda.gov/opacom/laws (accessed 20 March 2009).

Felli, J.C., Noel, R.A. and Cavazzoni, P.A. (2008) A multiattribute model for evaluating the benefit–risk profiles of treatment alternatives. *Medical Decision Making*, **29**, 104–15.

Fitzgerald, J.D. (1987) Clinical benefits, in *Medicines and Risk/Benefit Decisions* (eds S.R. Walker and A.W. Asscher), MTP Press Limited, Lancaster, pp. 127–34.

Food and Drug Administration (1988) CDER. Guideline for the format and content of the clinical and statistical sections of an application, July 1988. http://www.fda.gov/cder (accessed 20 March 2009).

Food and Drug Administration (1998) Guidance for industry; providing clinical evidence of effectiveness for human drug and biological products, FDA, May 1998. Available from http://www.fda.gov/cder (accessed 20 March 2009).

Food and Drug Administration (1999a) CDER Special Report. Benefit versus risk: how CDER approves new drugs. In: From test tube to patient: improving health through human drugs. Food and Drug Administration, FDA, 1999. Available from http://www.fda.gov/cder

Food and Drug Administration (1999b) Managing the risks from medical product use; creating a risk management framework. Report to the FDA Commissioner from the task force on risk management. FDA, 1999 May. http://www.fda.gov/cder (accessed 20 March 2009).

Food and Drug Administration (2001) Letter from J. Woodcock, Director of CDER, to consumers and health care providers, January 9 2001. http://www.fda.gov/cder (accessed 20 March 2009).

Food and Drug Administration (2002) CDER consumer information. Think it through: a guide to managing the benefits and risks of medicines FDA, 2002. http://www.fda.gov/cder (accessed 20 March 2009).

Food and Drug Administration (2003a). Concept paper; premarketing risk assessment [draft], 2003 March 3. http://www.fda.gov/cder (accessed 20 March 2009).

Food and Drug Administration (2003b) Concept paper; risk assessment of observational data: good pharmacovigilance practices and pharmacoepidemiologic assessment [draft], March 3 2003. http://www.fda.gov/cder (accessed 20 March 2009).

Food and Drug Administration (2004) Center for Drug Evaluation and Research. Manual of policies and procedures; clinical review template. http://www.fda.gov/cder (accessed 20 March 2009).

Friedman, M.A., Woodcock, J., Lumpkin, M.M., *et al.* (1999) The safety of newly approved medicines; do recent market removals mean there is a problem? *Journal of the American Medical Association*, **281**, 1728–34.

Galson, S. (2007) *Reducing the risks and increasing the benefits of marketed drugs – FDA response to the IOM report.* Presentation to the American College of Preventative Medicine, 24 February 2007. www.fda.gov/cder/present/galson/2007/ACPM022407FINAL.pdf (accessed March 23 2009).

Garratt, A., Schmidt, L., Mackintosh, A. and Fitzpatrick, R. (2002) Quality of life measurement: bibliographic study of patient assessed health outcome measures. *British Medical Journal*, **324**, 1417–21.

Garrison, L. (2007) *A structured health outcomes approach to the pre-marketing quantitative risk–benefit modeling of new pharmaceuticals.* Presented at the Benefit–risk Assessments for Drugs Workshop. Office of Health Economics, 24 October 2007, London, UK.

Garrison, L.P., Towse, A. and Bresnahan, B. (2007) Assessing a structured, quantitative health outcomes approach to drug risk-benefit analysis. *Health Affairs* **26**(3), 684–95.

Gelber, R.D., Cole, B.F., Gelber, S. and Goldhirsch, A. (1996) The Q-TwiST method, in *Quality of Life and Pharmacoeconomics in Clinical Trials* (ed. B. Spilker), Lippincott-Raven Publishers, Philadelphia, pp. 403–12.

Gift, T.L., Haddix, A.C. and Corso, P.S. (2003). Cost-effectiveness analysis, in *Prevention Effectiveness; a Guide to Decision Analysis and Economic Evaluation*, 2nd edn (eds A.C. Haddix, S.M. Teutsch and Corso P.S.), Oxford University Press, Oxford, pp. 156–77.

Gold, M.R., Siegel, J.E., *et al.* (1996) *Cost-effectiveness in health and medicine.* Oxford University Press, New York.

Greenhalgh, T. (1997) *How to read a paper; the basics of evidence based medicine.* BMJ Publishing Group, London.

Gruchalla, R.S. (2000) Clinical assessment of drug-induced disease. *Lancet*, **356**, 1505–11.

Guyatt, G.H., Sackett, D.L., Cook, D.J., for the evidence-based medicine working group (1993) Users' guide to the medical literature; II. How to use an article about therapy or prevention; A. are the results of the study valid? *Journal of the American Medical Asssociation*, **270**, 2598–601.

Guyatt, G.H., Sinclair, J., Cook, D.J. and Glasziou, P. (1999) Users' guide to the medical literature: XVI. How to use a treatment recommendation. *Journal of the American Medical Association*, **281**, 1836–43.

Hauber, A.B., Johnson, F.R. and Andrews, E.A. (2006) Risk-benefit analysis methods for pharmaceutical decision-making – where are we now? *ISPOR Connections*, **12**(6), 3–5.

Heeley, E., Waller, P. and Moseley, J. (2005) Testing and implementing signal impact analysis in a regulatory setting: results of a pilot study. *Drug Safety*, **28**(10), 901–6.

Herxheimer, A. (2001) Benefit, risk and harm. *Australian Prescriber*, **24**, 18.

Holden, W.L. (2003) Benefit–risk analysis: a brief review and proposed quantitative approaches. *Drug Safety*, **26**, 853–62.

Holden, W.L., Juhaeri, J. and Dai, W. (2003a) Benefit–risk analysis: a proposal using quantitative methods. *Pharmacoepidemiology and Drug Safety*, **12**, 611–16.

Holden, W.L., Juhaeri, J. and Dai, W. (2003b) Benefit–risk analysis: examples using quantitative methods. *Pharmacoepidemiology and Drug Safety*, **12**, 693–7.

Honig, P. (2007) Benefit and risk assessment in drug development and utilization: a role for clinical pharmacology. *Clinical Pharmacological Therapy*, **82**, 109–12.

Hughes, D.A., Bayoumi, A.M. and Pirmohamed, M. (2007) Current assessment of risk-benefit by regulators: is it time to introduce decision analysis. *Clinical Pharmacology & Therapeutics*, **82**, 123–7.

Hyslop, D.L., Read, H.A., Masica, D.N. and Kotsanos, J.G. (2002) Pharmaceutical risk management: a call to arms for pharmacoepidemiology. *Pharmacoepidemiology and Drug Safety*, **11**, 417–20.

Institute of Medicine. Drug safety report. September 2006, Washington DC.

International Conference on Harmonisation. *E9Statistical principles for clinical trials.* September 1998. http://www.fda.gov/cder/guidance/ICH_E9fnl.PDF

International Conference on Harmonisation (1995a) ICH topic E1A: Population exposure: the extent of population exposure to assess clinical safety, The European Medicines Evaluation Agency. http://www.emea.europa.eu (accessed 7 April 2009).

International Conference on Harmonisation (1995b) ICH topic E2A: Clinical safety data management: definitions and standards for expedited reporting, The European Medicines Evaluation Agency. http://www.emea.europa.eu (accessed 7 April 2009).

International Conference on Harmonisation (1996a) ICH topic E3: Structure and content of clinical study reports. The European Medicines Evaluation Agency. http://www.ich.org/cache/compo/475-272-1.html#E3 (accessed 6 April 2009).

International Conference on Harmonisation (1996b) ICH topic E6: Guideline for good clinical practice. The European Medicines Evaluation Agency.http://www.ich.org/cache/compo/475-272-1.html#E6 (accessed 6 April 2009)

International Conference on Harmonisation (1997) ICH topic E8: General considerations for clinical trials. The European Medicines Evaluation Agency. http://www.emea.europa.eu (accessed 7 April 2009).

International Conference on Harmonisation (1998) ICH topic E9: Statistical principles for clinical trials. The European Medicines Evaluation Agency. http://www.emea.europa.eu (accessed 7 April 2009).

International Conference on Harmonisation (2000) ICH topic M4: Common technical document for the registration of pharmaceuticals for human use. The European Medicines Evaluation Agency. http://www.emea.europa.eu (accessed 7 April 2009).

International Conference on Harmonisation (2004) [Homepage on the Internet]. Available from http://www.ich.org (accessed 20 March 2009).

Japan Pharmaceutical Manufacturers Association (2003) Pharmaceutical administration and regulations in Japan, JPMA. http://www.jpma.or.jp/index.html (accessed 20 March 2009).

Johnson, F.R. and Hauber, A.B. (2007) *Quantitative risk–benefit analysis for regulatory decision making: Alternatives and challenges.* Presented at the Benefit–risk Assessments for Drugs Workshop. Office of Health Economics, 24 October 2007, London, UK.

Johnson, F.R., Fillit, H., *et al.* (2007a) *Alzheimer's disease progression healthy-year equivalents: Stated risk–benefit trade-off preferences.* International Conference on Prevention of Dementia, Washington, DC. June 2007. http://www.rtihs.org/request/index.cfm?fuseaction=display&PID=9517 (accessed 23 March 2009).

Johnson, F.R., Ozdemir, S. *et al.* (2007b) Women's willingness to accept perceived risks for vasomotor symptom relief. *Journal of Womens Health*, **16**(7), 1028–40.

Johnson, N., Lilford, R.J., Mayers, D., *et al*. (1994) Do healthy asymptomatic postmenopausal women with a uterus want routine cyclical hormone replacement? A utility analysis. *Journal of Obstetrics and Gynaecology*, **14**, 35–9.

Johnson, F.R., Ozdemir, S., Mansfield, C., *et al*. (2007) Crohn's disease patients' risk–benefit preferences: serious adverse event risks versus treatment efficacy. *Gastroenterology*, **133**(3), 769–79.

Jones, R. (2002) Efficacy and safety of COX 2 inhibitors. *British Medical Journal*, **325**, 607–8.

Kaufman, D.W. and Shapiro, S. (2000) Epidemiological assessment of drug induced disease. *Lancet*, **356**, 1339–43.

Keeney, R.L. (1992) *Value-Focused Thinking: a Path to Creative Decision-Making*, Harvard University Press, Cambridge, MA, USA.

Keeney, R.L. and Raiffa, H. (1976) Decisions with multiple objectives, John Wiley & Sons, New York.

Kessler, D.A., Pape, S.M. and Sundwall, D.N. (1987) The Federal regulation of medical devices. *New England Journal of Medicine*, **317**, 357–66.

Kirkwood, C.W. (1996) *Strategic Decision Making: Multiobjective Decision Analysis with Spreadsheets*, Wadsworth Publishing Co, Belmont, CA, USA, 1996.

Konstam, M. (2003) Matters of the heart: assessing the cardiovascular safety of new drugs. *American Heart Journal*, **146**, 561–2.

Kruse, W., Eggert-Kruse, W., Rampmaier, J., *et al*. (1991) Dosage frequency and drug compliance behaviour; a comparative study on compliance with a medication to be taken twice or four times daily. *European Journal of Clinical Pharmacology*, **41**, 589–92.

Lasagna, L. (1998) Balancing risks versus benefits in drug therapy decisions. *Clinical Therapeutics*, **20**, C72–C79.

Lasser, K.E., Allen, P.D., Woolhandler, S.J., *et al*. (2002) Timing of new black box warnings and withdrawals for prescription medications. *Journal of the American Medical Association*, **287**, 2215–20.

Laupacis, A., Sackett, D.L. and Roberts, R.S. (1988) An assessment of clinically useful measures of the consequences of treatment. *New England Journal of Medicine*, **318**(26), 1728–33.

Lebow, M.A. (1999) The pill and the press: reporting risk. *Obstetrics & Gynecology*, **93**, 453–6.

Lee, T.R. (1987) The risks in society, in *Medicines and Risk/Benefit Decisions* (eds S.R. Walker and A.W. Asscher), MTP Press Limited, Lancaster, pp. 5–12.

Lehner, J.P., Meyer, F., Juillet, Y., les participants à la table ronde no. 1 de Giens XVI (2001) Communication et transparence de l'évaluation du risque et bénéfice en santé publique: exemple du médicament. *Thérapie*, **56**, 335–9.

Lewis, J.H. (1993) Risk/benefit assessment of new drugs: perspectives of a former FDA Advisory Committee member. *Drug Information Journal*, **27**, 1037–49.

Lilford, R.J. and Braunholtz, D. (1996) For debate: the statistical basis for public policy: a paradigm shift is overdue. *British Medical Journal*, **313**, 603–7.

Lilford, R.J. and Jackson, J. (1995) Equipoise and the ethics of randomisation. *Journal of the Royal Society of Medicine*, **88**, 552–9.

Lilford, R.J., Pauker, S.G., Braunholtz, D.A. and Chard, J. (1998) Decision analysis and the implementation of research findings. *British Medical Journal*, **317**, 405–9.

Llewellyn-Thomas, H.A., Williams, J.I., Levy, L. and Naylor, C.D. (1996) Using a trade-off technique to assess patients' treatment preferences for benign prostatic hyperplasia. *Medical Decision Making*, **16**, 262–72.

Localio, A.R., Margolis, D.J. and Berlin, J.A. (2007) Relative risks and confidence intervals were easily computed indirectly from multivariable logistic regression. *Journal of Clinical Epidemiology*, **60**, 874–82.

Loke, Y.K., Bell, A. and Derry, S. (2003) Aspirin for the prevention of cardiovascular disease: calculating benefit and harm in the individual patient. *British Journal of Clinical Pharmacology*, **55**, 282–7.

Lumpkin, M.M. (2000) International pharmacovigilance: developing cooperation to meet the challenges of the 21st century. *Pharmacology & Toxicology*, **86** (Suppl I), 20–2.

Lynd, L.D. (2007a) An example of incremental net benefit analysis using Lotronex, in Drug Information Association 43rd Annual Meeting, 2007, Atlanta, USA.

Lynd, L.D. (2007b) Using incremental net benefit for quantitative benefit–risk analysis – Case studies of Vioxx and Lotronex. Presented at the Benefit–risk Assessments for Drugs Workshop. Office of Health Economics, 24 October 2007, London, UK.

Lynd, L.D. and O'Brien, B.J. (2004) Advances in risk benefit evaluation using probabilistic simulation methods: an application to the prophylaxis of deep vein thrombosis. *Journal of Clinical Epidemiology*, **57**, 795–803.

MacGregor, A.D. and Perry, W.L. (1962) Detection of drug toxicity. *Lancet*, **1**, 1233.

McGregor, M. and Caro, J.J. (2006) QALYs: are they helpful to decision makers? *Pharmacoeconomics*, **24**(10), 947–52.

Mancini, G.B.J. and Schulzer, M. (1999) Reporting risks and benefits of therapy by use of the concepts of unqualified success and unmitigated failure: applications to highly cited trials in cardiovascular medicine. *Circulation*, **99**, 377–83.

Martin, A.J., Lumley, T.S. and Simes, R.J. (1996) Incorporating trade-offs in quality of life assessment, in *Quality of Life and Pharmacoeconomics in Clinical Trials* (ed. B. Spilker), Lippincott-Raven Publishers, Philadelphia, pp. 403–12.

Martindale (2002) *The Complete Drug Reference*, 33th edn (ed. S.C. Sweetman), Pharmaceutical Press, London.

Marwick, C. (1999) Drug safety takes cooperation. *Journal of the American Medical Association*, **282**, 315–*16*.

Matheson, D. and Matheson, J. (1998) *The Smart Organization: Creating Value Through Strategic R&D*. Harvard Business School Press, Boston.

Medicines Evaluation Board (1999) Public assessment report Maxalt. Available from http://www. cbg-meb.nl/CBG/en/human-medicines/actueel/1999-03-01-Public+Assessment+Report+of+ the+Medicines+Evaluation+Board+Rizatriptan+Maxalt/default.htm (accessed 6 April 2009).

Meiners, A.P. (2002) *Transparency and communication of the benefit–risk assessment, patients' expectations [presentation], Drug Information Association Annual Euromeeting 2002*, Basel, Switzerland, March 6, 2002. http://www.diahome.org (accessed 20 March 2009).

Messonnier, M. and Meltzer, M. (2003) *Cost-benefit analysis, in Prevention Effectiveness: a Guide to Decision Analysis and Economic Evaluation*, 2nd edn (eds A.C. Haddix, S.M. Teutsch and P.S. Corso), Oxford University Press, Oxford, pp. 127–55.

Meyboom, R.H.B. and Egberts, A.C.G. (1999) Comparing therapeutic benefit and risk. *Thérapie*, **54**, 29–34.

Miller, L.L. (1992) Pitfalls in the drug approval process: dose-effect, experimental design, and risk-benefit issues. *Drug Information Journal*, **26**, 251–60.

Miller, L.L. (1993) Risk/benefit assessment: the 'greased pig' of drug development. *Drug Information Journal*, **27**, 1011–20.

Moher, D., Schulz, K.F., Altman, D.G., for the CONSORT group (2001) The CONSORT statement: revised recommendations for improving the quality of reports of parallel-group randomised trials. *Lancet*, **357**, 1191–4.

Moynihan, R., Bero, L., Ross-Degnan, D., *et al.* (2000) Coverage by the news media of the benefits and risks of medications. *New England Journal of Medicine*, **342**, 1645–50.

Mussen, F. (2001) Balancing risks and benefits – science or opinions [unpublished communication]. Management Forum seminar (in association with the Medicines Control Agency) *'Risk Benefit Assessment'*, November 8, 2001, London.

Mussen, F. (2002) Balancing risks and benefits – science or opinions [unpublished communication]. *Management Forum seminar 'Benefit Risk Assessment'*, November 29, 2002, London.

Mussen, F. (2005) The evaluation of methods for benefit risk assessment of medicines and the development of a new model using multi criteria decision analysis. Doctoral Thesis, University of Wales.

Mussen, F., Salek, S. and Walker, S. (2007) A quantitative approach to benefit–risk assessment of medicines – part 1: the development of a new model using multi-criteria decision analysis. *Pharmacoepidemiology and Drug Safety*, **16**, S2–S15.

Naimark, D., Krahn, M.D., Naglie, G., *et al.* (1997) Primer on medical decision analysis: part 5 – working with Markov processes. *Medical Decision Making*, **17**, 152–59.

Naito, C. (1994) Evaluation methods for clinical trials of drugs in Japan which may affect ethnic differences, in *The Relevance of Ethnic Factors in the Clinical Evaluation of Medicines* (ed. S. Walker), Kluwer Academic, Boston, pp. 49–62.

National Institute for Clinical Excellence (2004) *Guide to the methods of technology appraisal.* April 2004, NICE, London.

Naylor, C.D. and Llewellyn-Thomas, H.A. (1994) Can there be a more patient-centred approach to determining clinically important effect sizes for randomised treatment trials? *Journal of Clinical Epidemiology*, **47**, 787–95.

Official Journal of the European Communities (2004) Directive 2001/83/EC of the European Parliament and of the Council of 6 November 2001 on the Community code relating to medicinal products for human use, Official Journal L 136, 30/04/2004, 34–84.

O'Neill, R. (2008) A perspective on characterizing benefits and risks derived from clinical trials: can we do more? *Drug Information Journal*, **42**, 235–44.

PatientView (2002) EU patients do not trust doctors and pharmacists to give satisfactory information on prescribing drugs [press release], 2002 June. http://www.patient-view.com (accessed 20 March 2009).

Patten, S.B. and Lee, R.C. (2002) Modeling methods for facilitating decisions in pharmaceutical policy and population therapeutics. *Pharmacoepidemiology and Drug Safety*, **11**, 165–8.

Pearce, L.B., Pitman, A., Greenburg, A.G., *et al.* (2008) Application of a unique scoring system for numerical determination of a benefit risk ratio in clinical trials. *Clinical Pharmacology & Therapeutics*, **83**, S87–S88.

Penfornis, A. (2003) Observance médicamenteuse dans le diabète de type 2: influence des modalités du traitement médicamenteux et conséquences sur son éfficacité. *Diabetes & Metabolism*, **29** (suppl), S31–S37.

Perfetto, E.M., Ellison, R., Ackermann, S., *et al.* (2003) Evidence-based risk management: how can we succeed? Deliberations from a risk management advisory council. *Drug Information Journal*, **37**, 127–34.

Phillips, L. (2007) *Multi-criteria decision analysis*. Presented at the Benefit–risk Assessments for Drugs Workshop, Office of Health Economics, 24 October 2007, London, UK.

Phillips, L.D. and Costa, C.A.B. (2007) Transparent prioritisation, budgeting and resource allocation with multi-criteria decision analysis and decision conferencing. *Annals of Operations Research*, **154**(1), 51–68.

Physicians' Desk Reference (2008) PDR Electronic Library, The Thomson Corporation.

Piantadosi, S. (1995) David Byar as a teacher. *Controlled Clinical Trials*, **16**, 202–11.

Pignatti, F., Aronsson, B., Vamvakas, S., *et al.* (2002) Clinical trials for registration in the European Union: the EMEA 5-year experience in oncology. *Critical Reviews in Oncology/ Hematology*, **42**, 123–35.

Pitt, B., Poole-Wilson, P., Segal, R., *et al* (2000) Effect of losartan compared with captopril on mortality in patients with symptomatic heart failure: randomised trial – the losartan heart failure survival study ELITE II. *Lancet*, **355**, 1582–7.

Pocock, S.J. (1996) *Clinical Trials: a Practical Approach*, John Wiley & Sons, Chichester.

Pritchett, Y.L. and Tamura, R. (2007) Global benefit–risk assessment in designing clinical trials and some statistical considerations of the method. *Pharmaceutical Statistics*, **7**, 170–8.

Puliyel, J.M. (2002) The dummies' guide to risk-benefit analysis of vaccines. Pediatrics, **110**, 193.

Rawlins, M.D. (1987) Risk-benefit decisions in licensing changes, in *Medicines and Risk/Benefit Decisions* (eds S.R. Walker and A.W. Asscher), MTP Press Limited, Lancaster, pp. 137–41.

Rawlins, M.D. (1995) Pharmacovigilance: paradise lost, regained or postponed? *Journal of the Royal College of Physicians of London*, **29**, 41–9.

Risk:benefit analysis of drugs in practice; the doctor the patient and the licensing authority (1995). *Drug and Therapeutics Bulletin*, **33**, 33–5.

Rothenberg, M.L., Carbone, D.P. and Johnson, D.H. (2003) Improving the evaluation of new cancer treatments: challenges and opportunities. *Nature Reviews – Cancer*, **3**, 303–9.

Sawaya, G.F., Guirguis-Blake, J., LeFevre, *et al.*, for the US Preventive Services Task Force (2007) Update on the methods of the US Preventive Services Task Force: estimating certainty and magnitude of net benefit. *Annals of Internal Medicine*, **147**, 871–5.

Slovic, P. (1987) Perception of risk. *Science*, **236**, 280–5.

Schiller, L.R. and Johnson, D.A. (2008) Balancing drug risk and benefit: toward refining the process of FDA decisions affecting patient care. *American Journal of Gastroenterology*, **103**, 815–19.

Schosser, R. (2002) Risk/benefit evaluation of drugs: the role of the pharmaceutical industry in Germany. *European Surgical Research*, **34**, 203–7.

SCRIP (2000) Rezulin was 'outmoded', says FDA, *SCRIP*, **2542**, 20.

Shaffer, M.L. and Watterberg, K.L. (2006) Joint distribution approaches to simultaneously quantifying benefit and risk. *BMC Medical Research Methodology*, **6**, 48.

Shakespeare, T.P., Gebski, V.J., Veness, M.J. and Simes, J. (2001) Improving interpretation of clinical studies by use of confidence levels, clinical significance curves, and risk-benefit contours. *Lancet*, **357**, 1349–53.

Simon, L.S. (2002) Pharmacovigilance: towards a better understanding of the benefit to risk ratio. *Annals of the Rheumatic Diseases*, **61** (suppl II), ii88–ii89.

Skolbekken, J.-A. (1998) Communicating the risk reduction achieved by cholesterol reducing drugs. *British Medical Journal*, **316**, 1956–8.

Slovic, P. (1987) Perception of risk. *Science*, **236**, 280–5.

Smeeth, L., Haines, A. and Ebrahim, S. (1999) Numbers needed to treat derived from meta-analyses – sometimes informative, usually misleading. *British Medical Journal*, **318**, 1548–51.

Smith, G.D. and Egger, M. (1994) Who benefits from medical interventions? *British Medical Journal*, **308**, 72–4.

Spilker, B. (1994) Incorporating benefit-to-risk determinations in medicine development. *Drug News & Perspectives*, **7**, 53–9.

Swales, J.D. (1997) Science in a health service. *Lancet*, **349**, 1319–21.

Tan, L.B. and Murphy, R. (1999) Shifts in mortality curves: saving or extending lives? *Lancet*, **354**, 1378–81.

Taylor, R.S., Drummond, M.F., Salkeld, G. and Sullivan, S.D. (2004) Inclusion of cost effectiveness in licensing requirements of new drugs: the fourth hurdle. *British Medical Journal*, **329**, 972–5.

Temple, R.J. and Himmel, M.H. (1999) Safety of newly approved drugs: implications for prescribing. *Journal of the American Medical Association*, **287**, 2273–5.

Temple, R. (2007) Quantitative decision analysis: a work in progress. *Clinical Pharmacology & Therapeutics*, **82**, 127–30.

The School of Community, Health Sciences and Social Care (2000) *Validity*. University of Salford. http://www.chssc.salford.ac.uk/healthSci/resmeth2000/remeth/validity.htm (accessed 22 March 2009).

The SOLVD Investigators (1991) Effect of enalapril on survival in patients with reduced left ventricular ejection fractions and congestive heart failure. *New England Journal of Medicine*, **325**, 193–302.

The Uppsala Monitoring Centre (2002a) Benefit, harm, effectiveness and risk in medicine, in *Viewpoint part I*. WHO Collaborating Centre for International Drug Monitoring, Uppsala.

The Uppsala Monitoring Centre (2002b) The risks of being alive, in *Viewpoint part I*. WHO Collaborating Centre for International Drug Monitoring, Uppsala.

Thompson, I.M., Klein, E.A., Lippman, S.M., *et al.* (2003) Prevention of prostate cancer with finasteride: A US/European perspective. *European Urology*, **44**, 650–5.

Troche, C.J., Paltiel, A.D. and Makuch, R.W. (2000) Evaluation of therapeutic strategies: a new method for balancing benefit and risk. *Value in Health*, **3**, 12–22.

Urquhart, J. (2001) Mis- and non-use of prescription drugs: confusion, lost revenues and future commercial opportunities. *Pharmaceutical Visions*, summer, 9–17.

Valuck, R.J., Libby, A.M., *et al.* Spillover effects on treatment of adult depression in primary care after FDA advisory on risk of pediatric suicidality with selective serotonin reuptake inhibitors. *American Journal of Psychiatry*, **164**(8), 1198–205.

VanTrigt, A.M., De Jong-Van DenBerg, L.T.W., Voogt, L.M., *et al.* (1995) Setting the agenda: does the medical literature set the agenda for articles about medicines in the newspapers? *Social Science & Medicine*, **41**, 893–9.

Veatch, R.M. (1993) Benefit/risk assessment: what patients can know that scientists cannot. *Drug Information Journal*, **27**, 1021–9.

Vioxx: an unequal partnership between safety and efficacy (2004) *Lancet*, **364**, 1287–8.

Walker, S.R. (1987) Introductory remarks, in *Medicines and Risk/Benefit Decisions* (eds S.R. Walker and A.W. Asscher), MTP Press Limited, Lancaster, pp. 1–2.

Waller, P. (2001) Pharmacoepidemiology – a tool for public health. *Pharmacoepidemiology and Drug Safety*, **10**, 165–72.

Walker, S. and Cone, M. (2004) Benefit–risk Assessment: Summary Report on the Workshop on the Development of a Model for Benefit–risk Assessment of Medicines Based on Multi-Criteria Decision Analysis. Centre for Medicines Research International, 2004, Surrey, UK.

Walker, S., Phillips, L.D., *et al*. Benefit–risk Assessment Model for Medicines: Developing a Structured Approach to Decision Making. Epsom: Centre for Medicines Research International, 2006, Surrey, UK.

Waller, P.C. and Evans, S.J.W. (2003) A model for the future conduct of pharmacovigilance. *Pharmacoepidemiology and Drug Safety*, **12**, 17–29.

Wardell, W.M. (1973) Therapeutic implications of the drug lag. *Clinical Pharmacology and Therapeutics*, **15**, 73–96.

Webster's Ninth New Collegiate Dictionary (1991) 9th edn. Merriam-Webster, Springfield.

Whitebrook, J. and Markey, J. (2008) *Industry and regulatory survey of benefit-risk management best practices*. Proceedings of the Drug Information Association Annual Meeting, Boston, USA, 2008, p. 89.

WHO Collaborating Centre for International Drug Monitoring (2004) Definitions [Internet page]. The Uppsala Monitoring Centre, WHO Collaborating Centre for International Drug Monitoring [updated 2004 October 11]. http://www.who-umc.org (accessed 7 April 2009).

Willan, A.R., O'Brien, B.J. and Cook, D.J. (1997) Benefit–risk ratios in the assessment of the clinical evidence of a new therapy. *Controlled Clinical Trials*, **18**, 121–30.

Wood, A.J.J. (1999) The safety of new medicines: the importance of asking the right questions. *Journal of the American Medical Association*, **281**, 1753–4.

World Health Organization (2003) *Adherence to Long-term Therapies: Evidence for Action*, World Health Organization, Geneva.

Index

Note: Figures and Tables are indicated by *italic page numbers*.

Benefit-Risk Appraisal of Medicines   Filip Mussen, Sam Salek, Stuart Walker
© 2009 John Wiley & Sons, Ltd

Index compiled by Paul Nash